WELCOME TO THE WONDERFUL WORLD OF RELAXING COLORATION

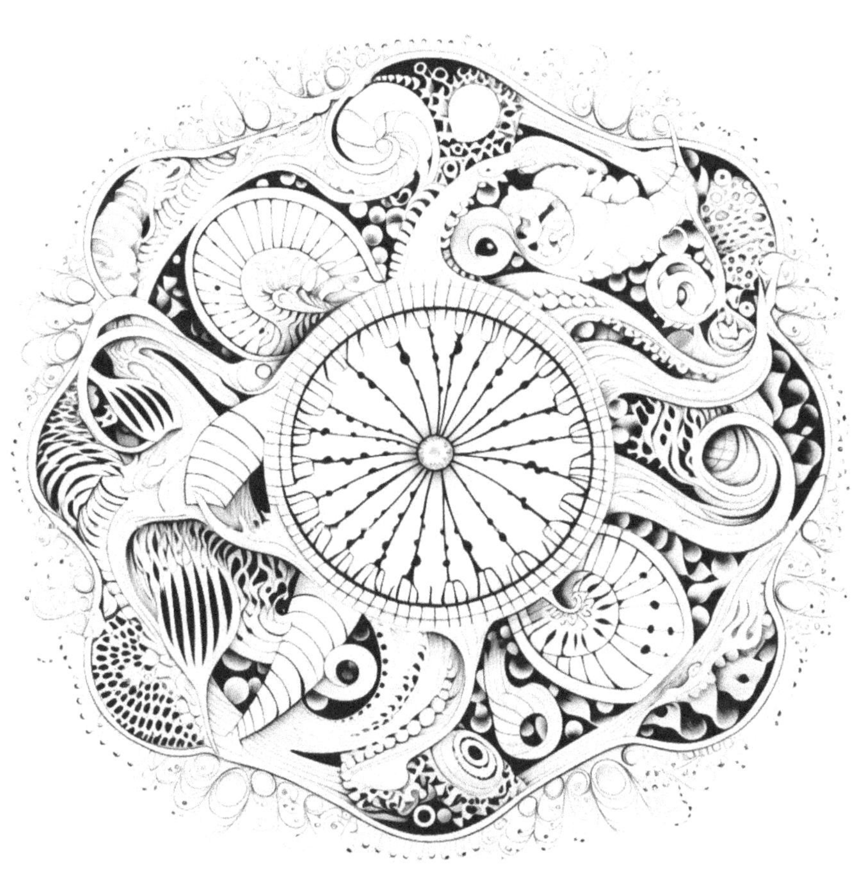

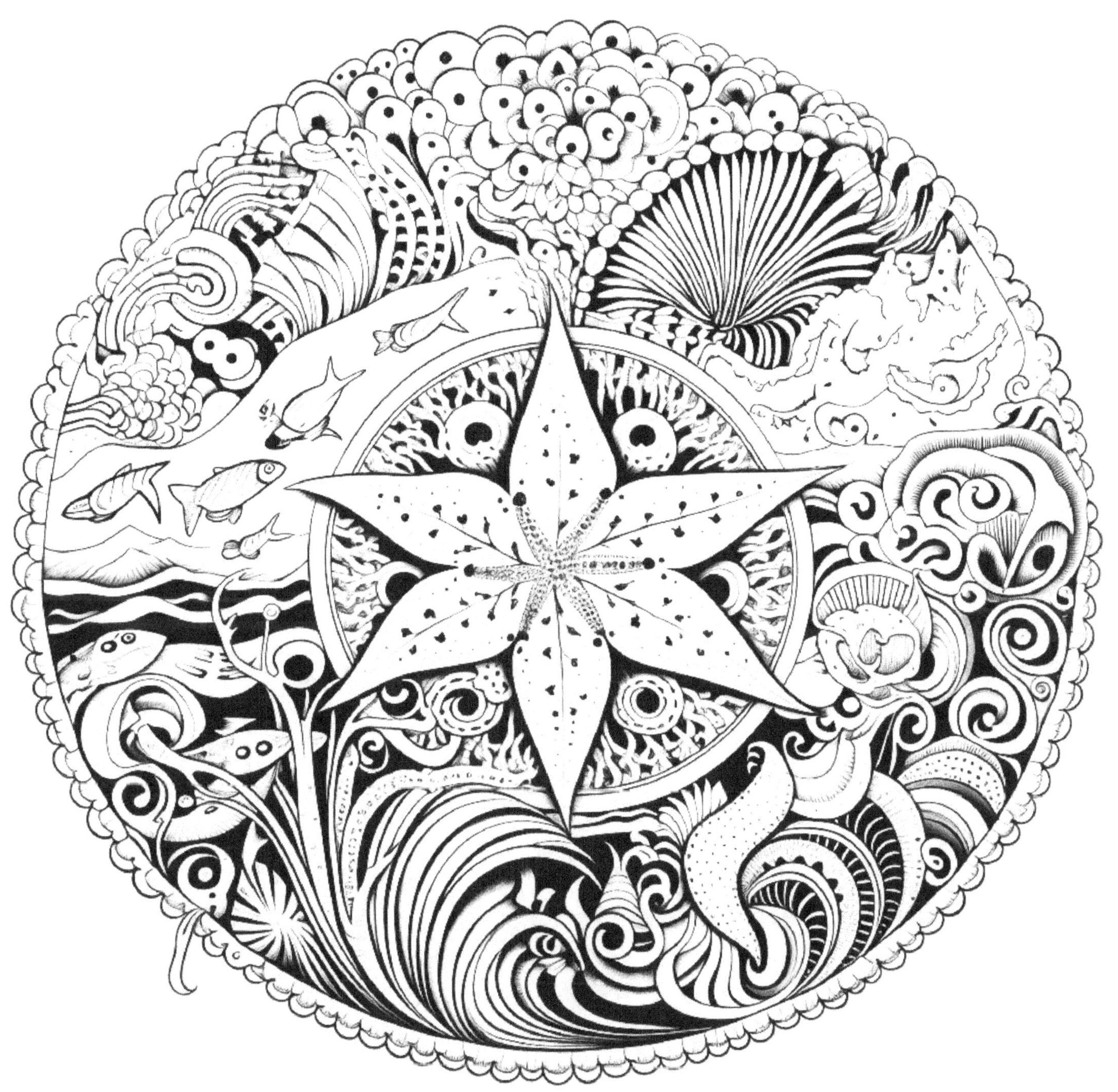

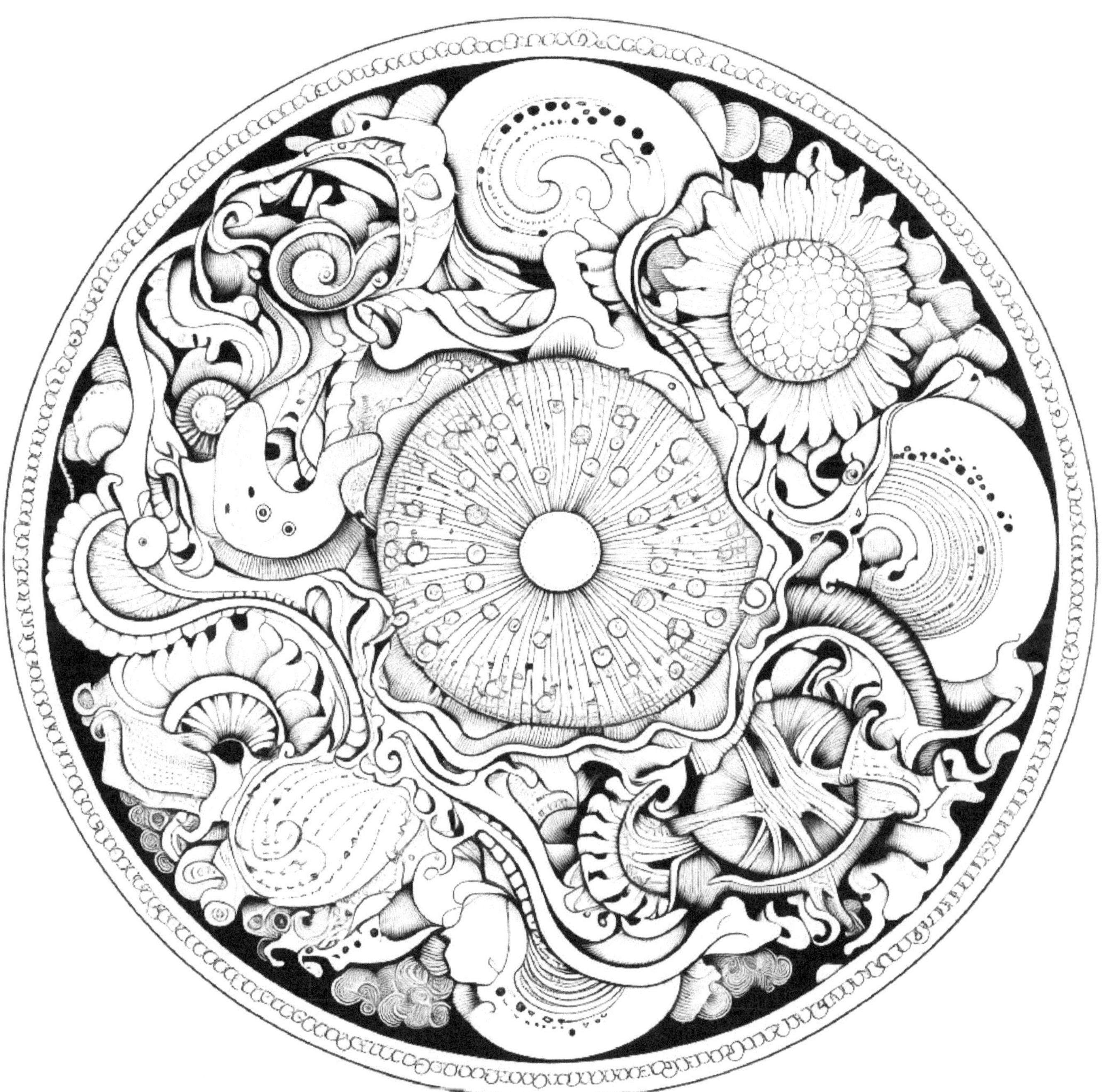

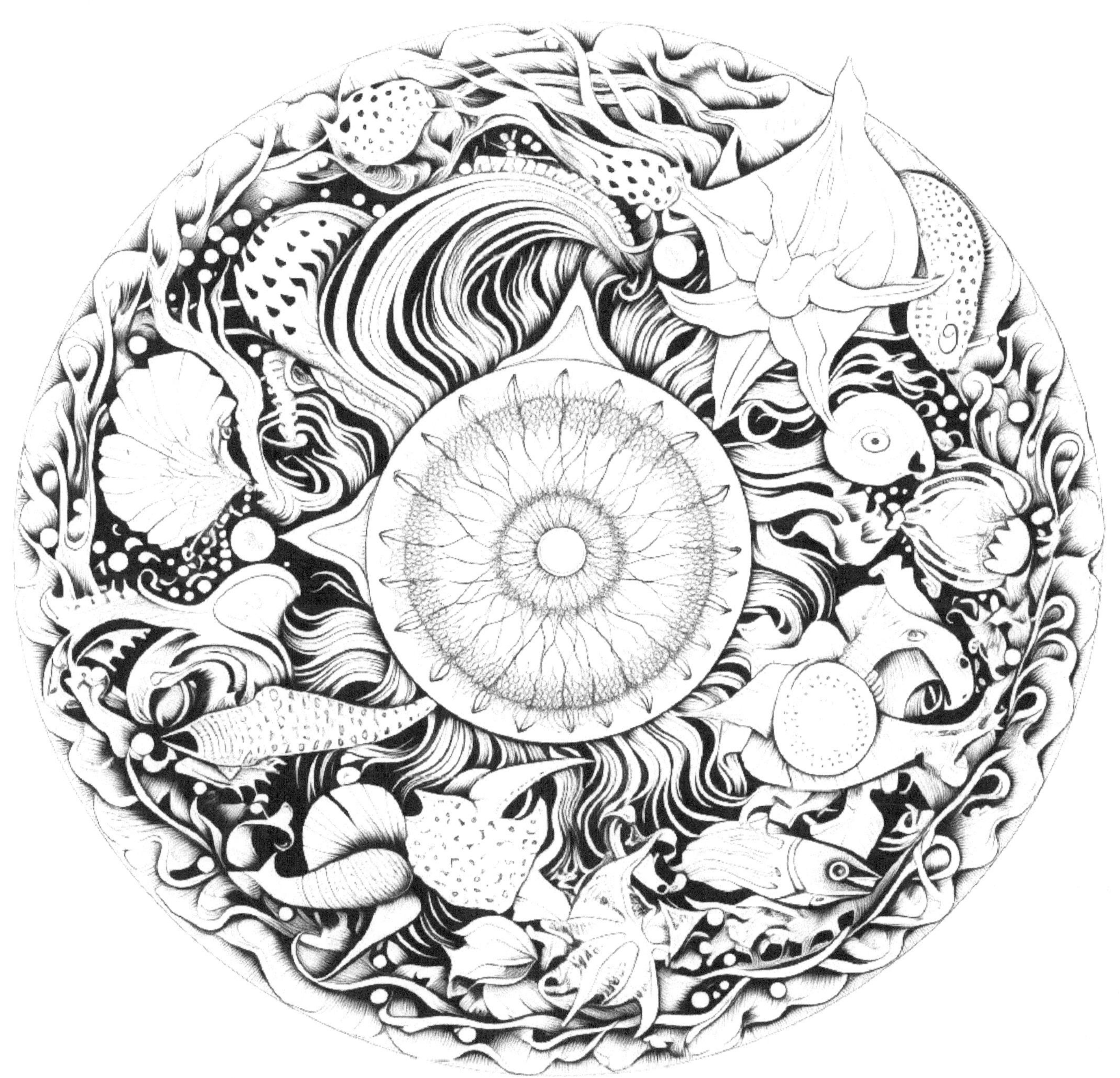

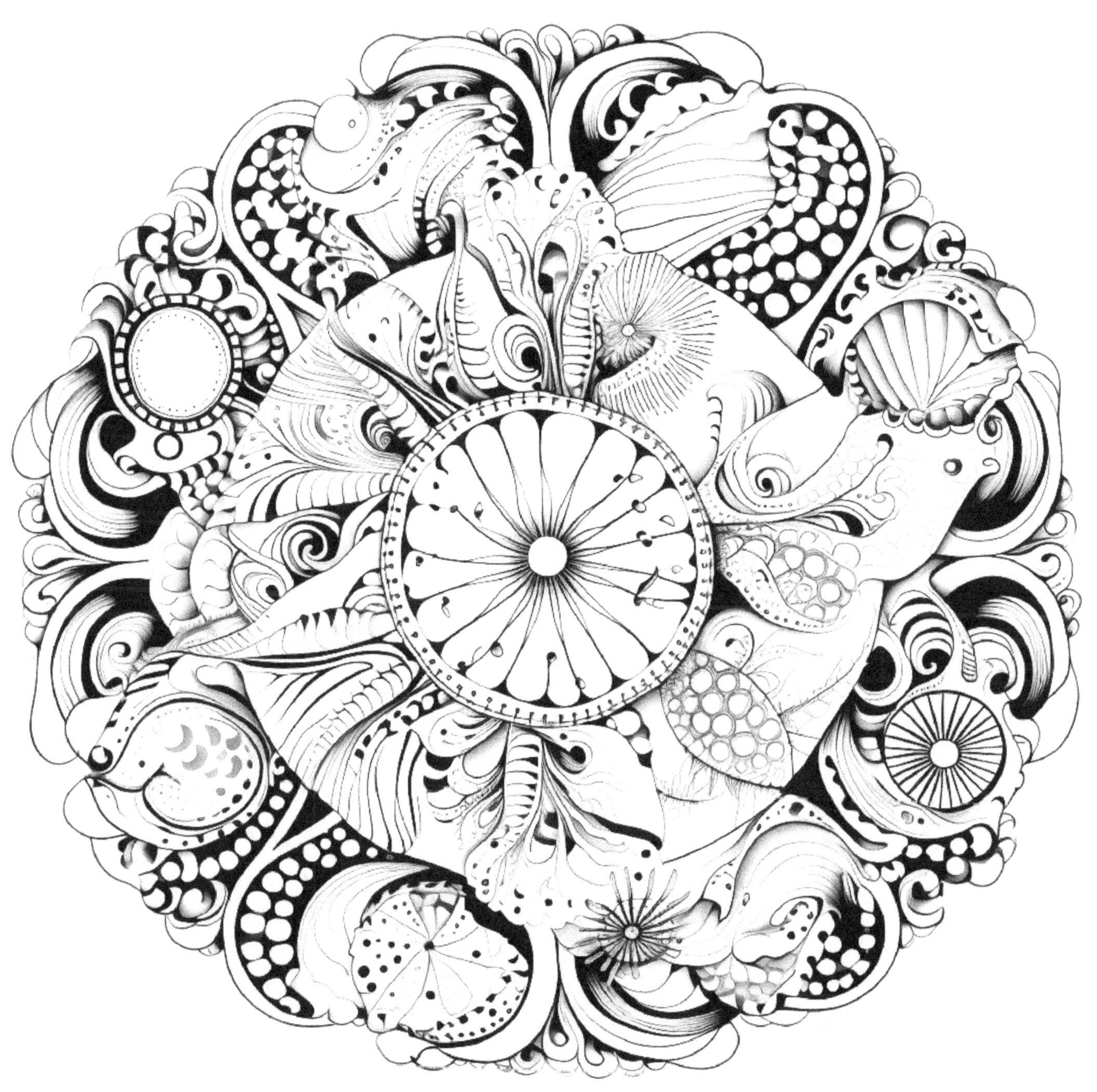

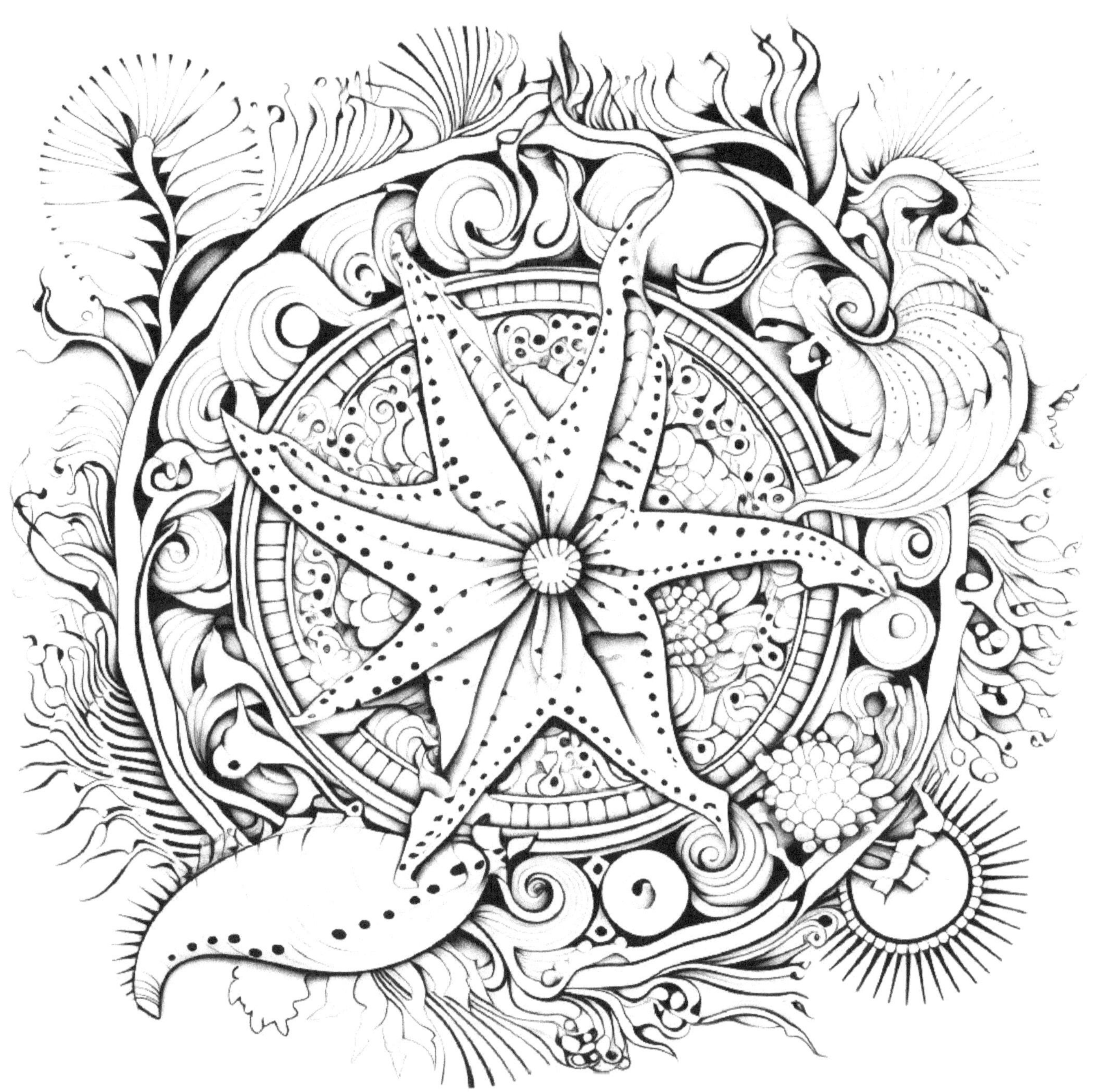

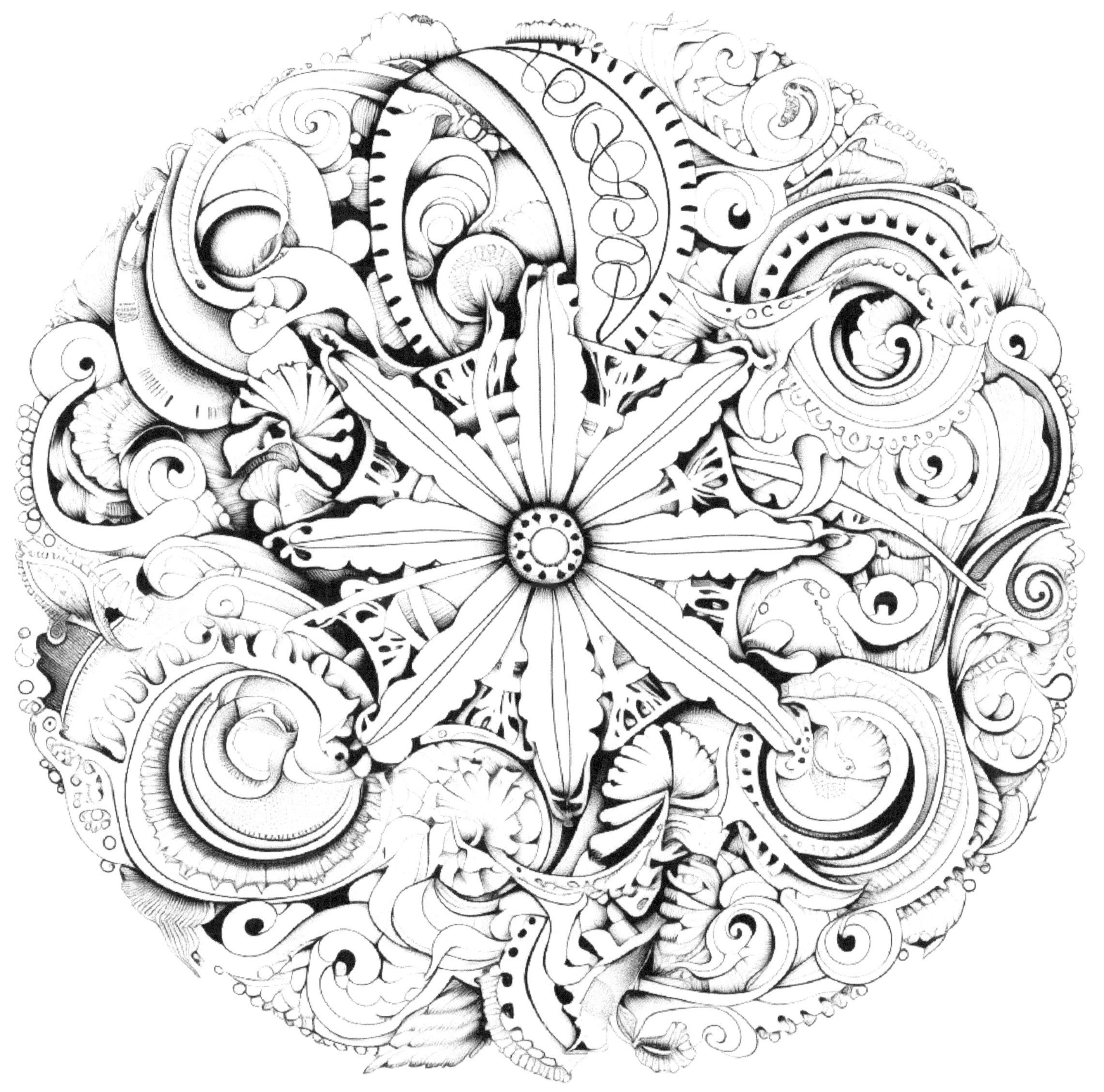

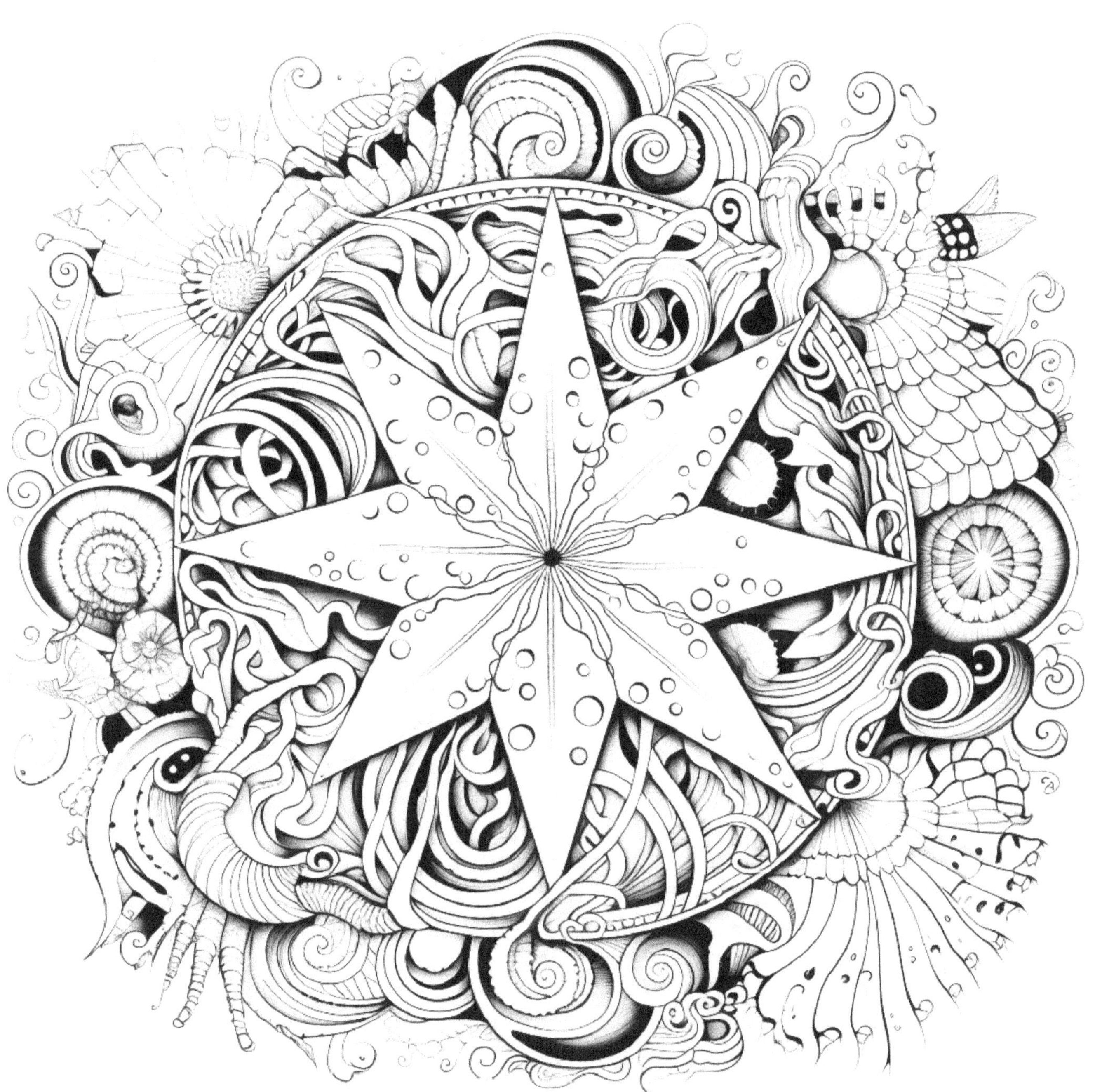

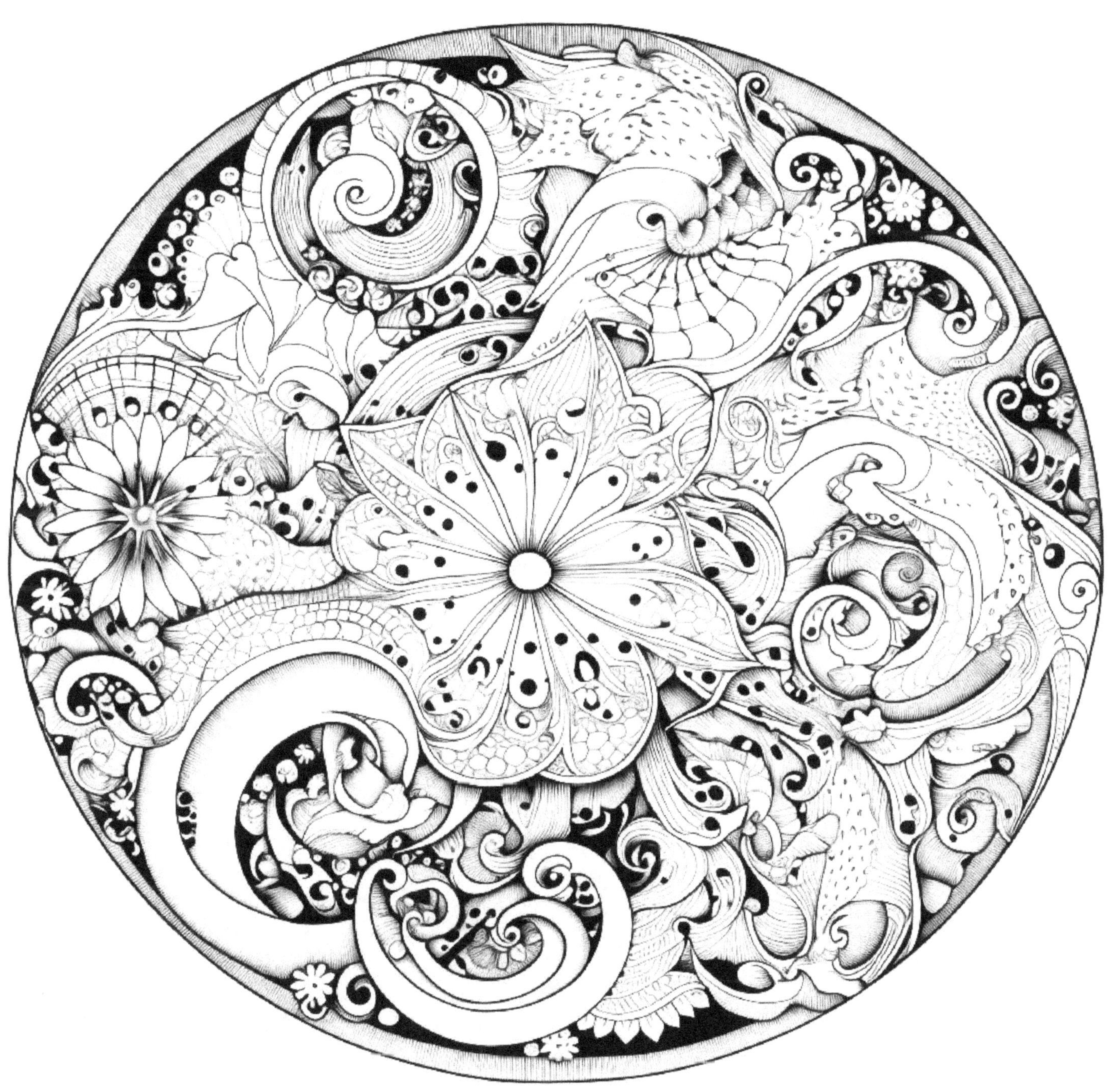

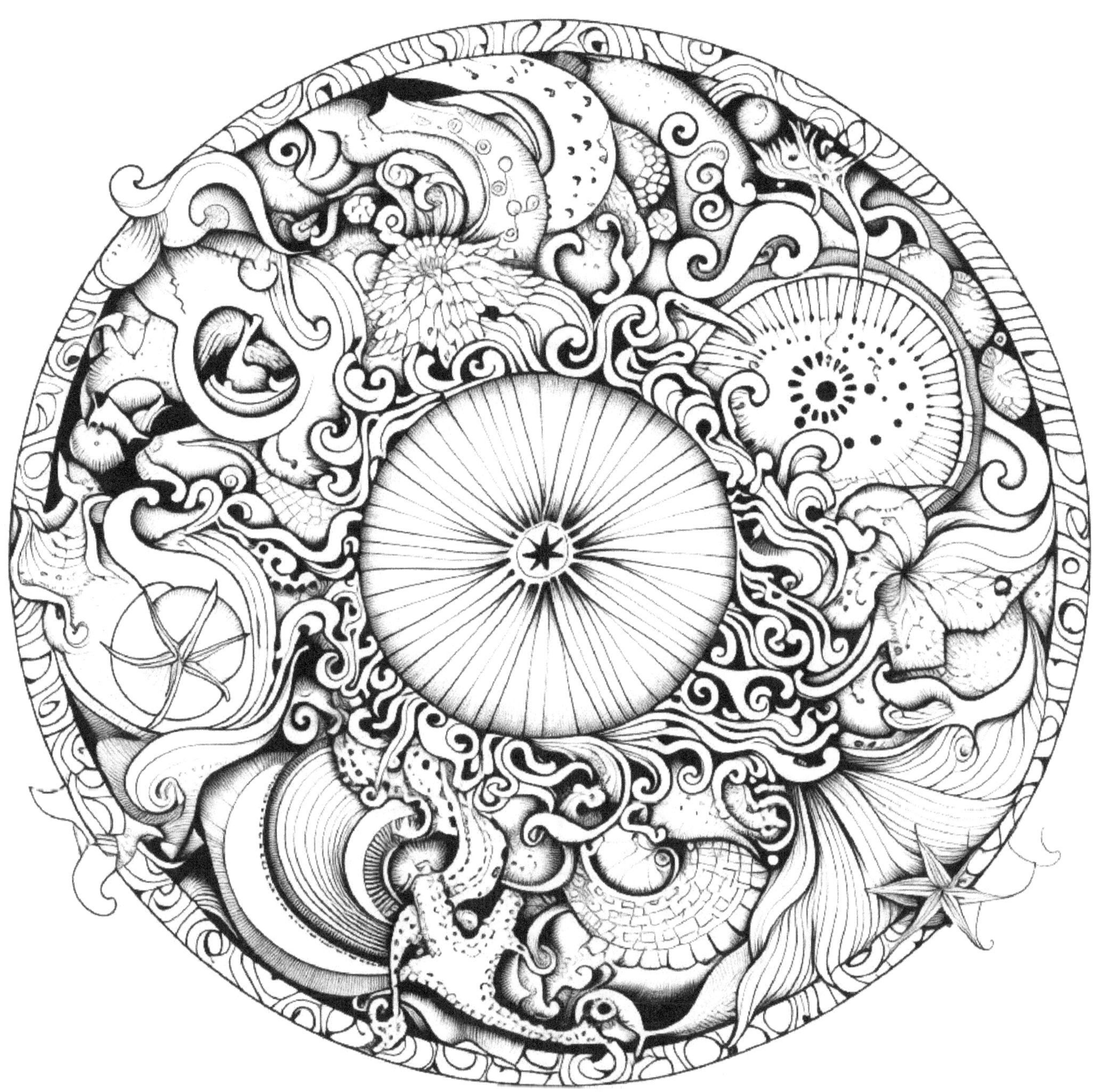

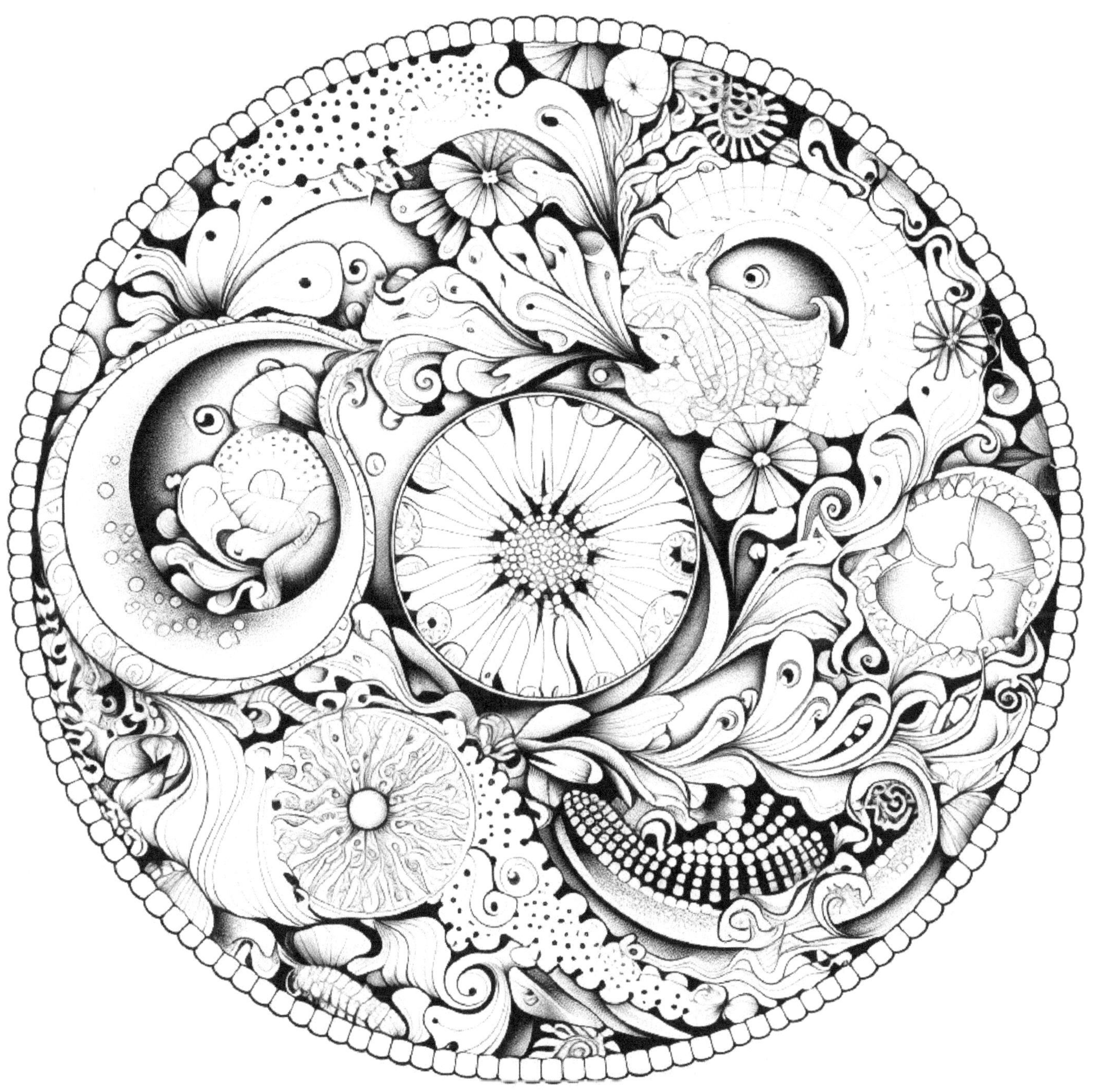

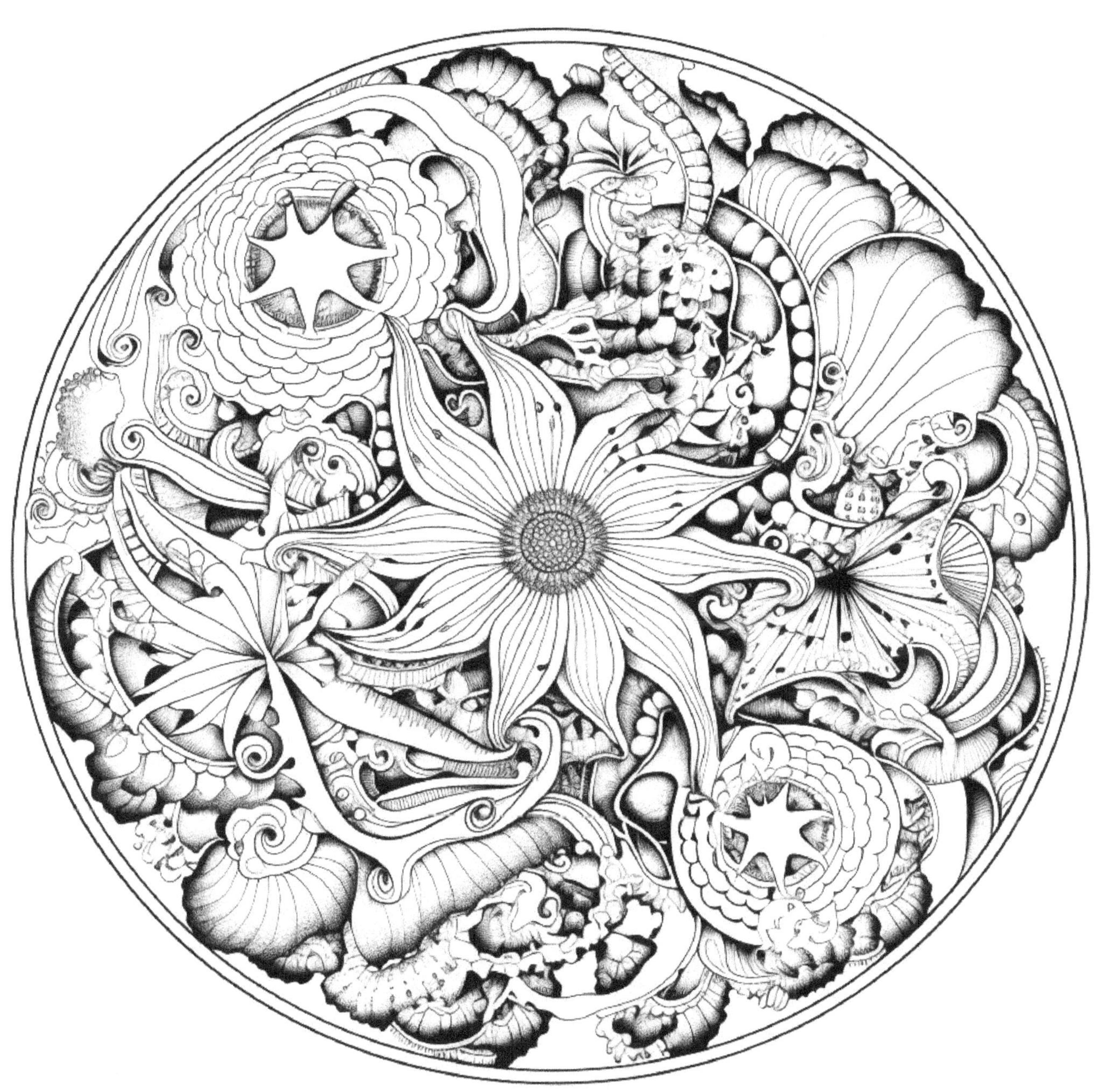

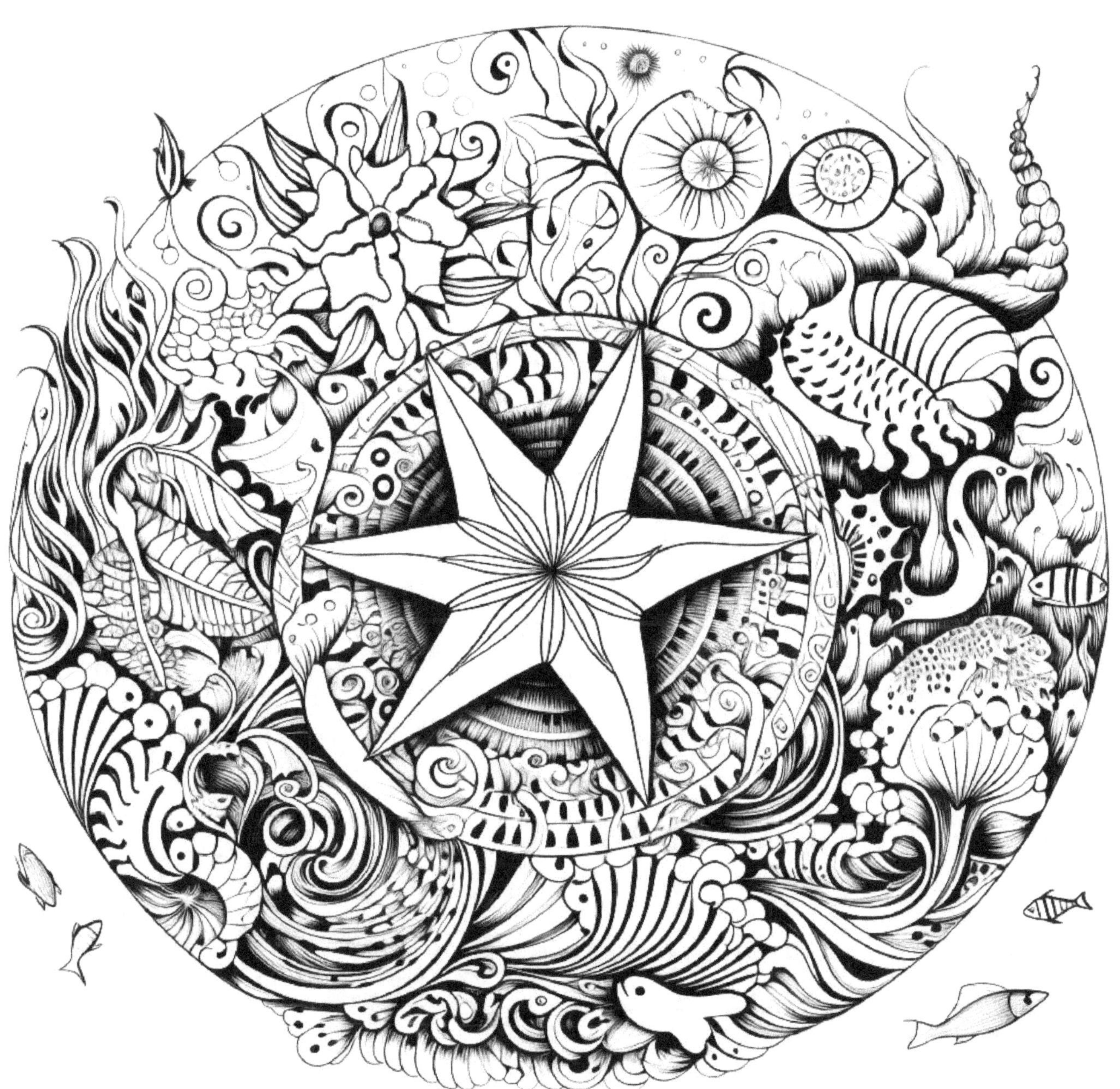

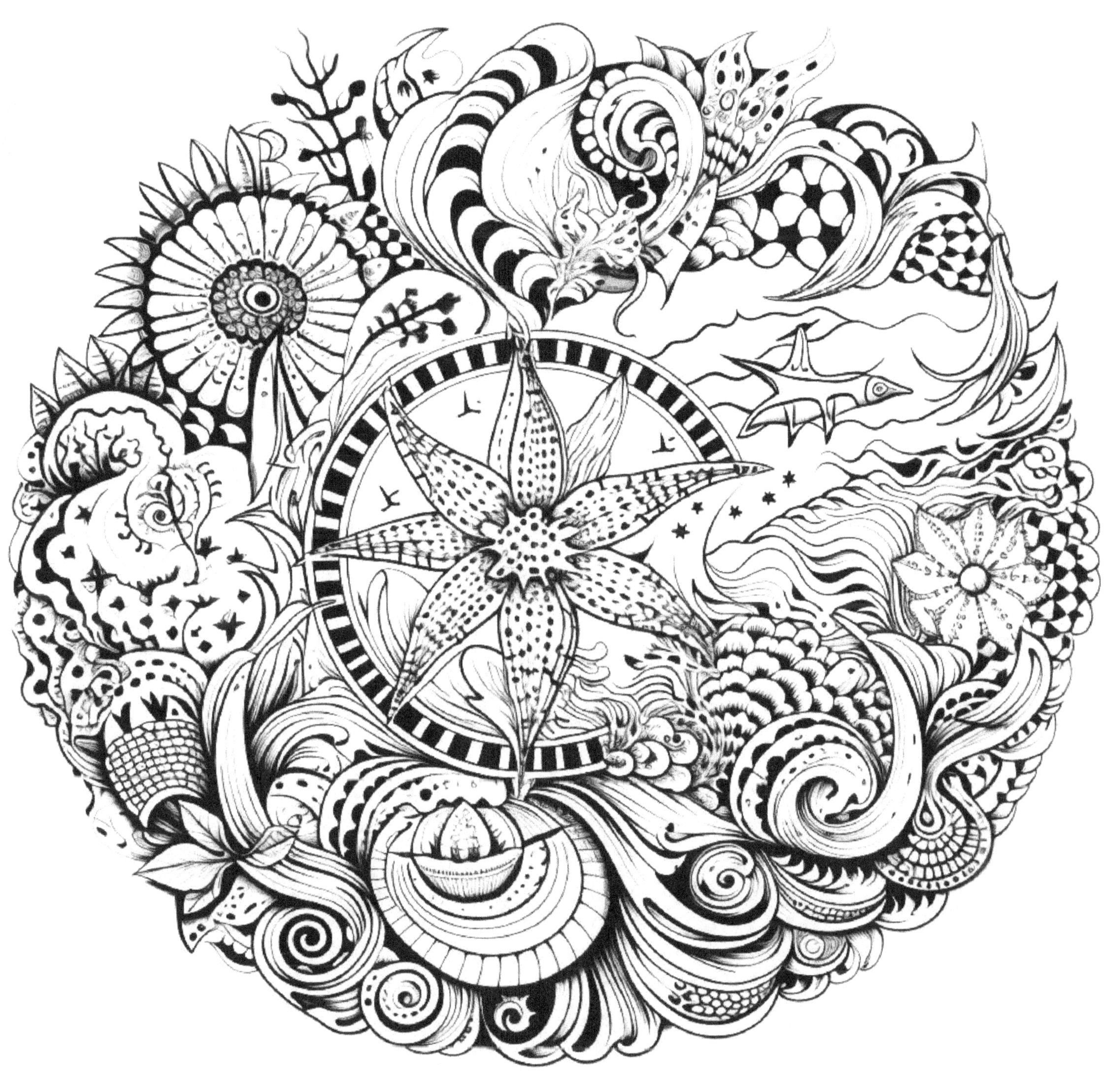

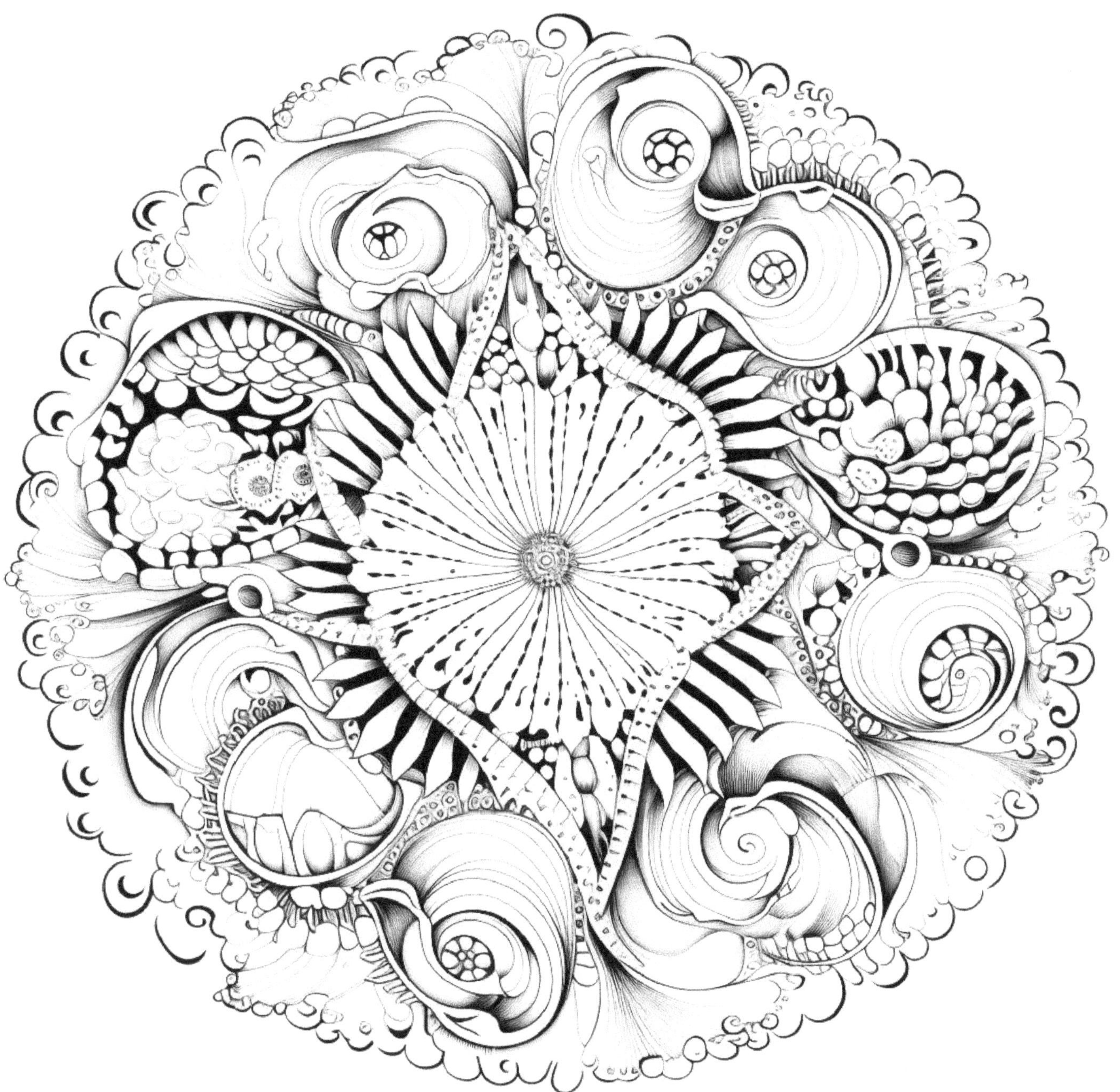

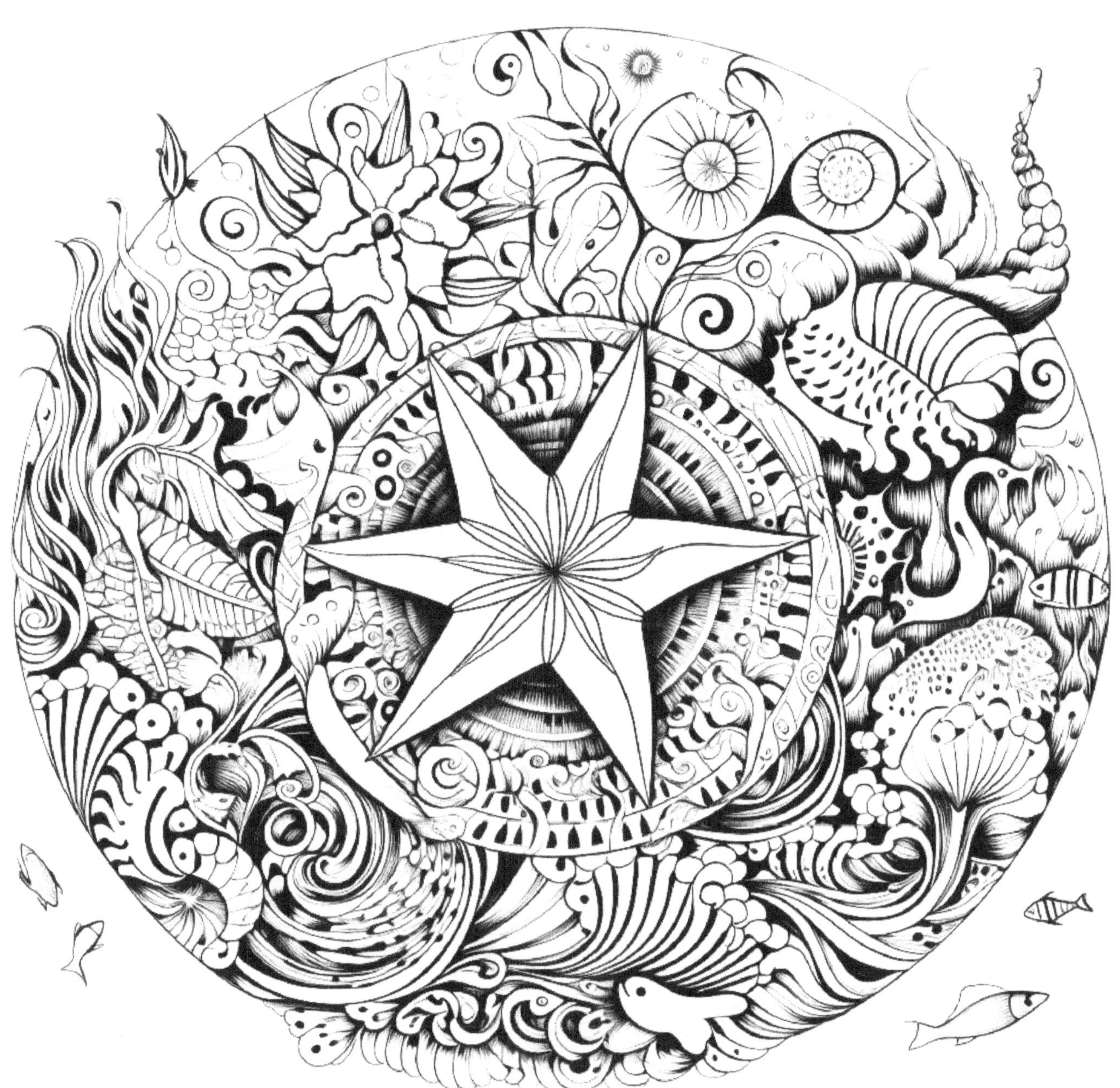

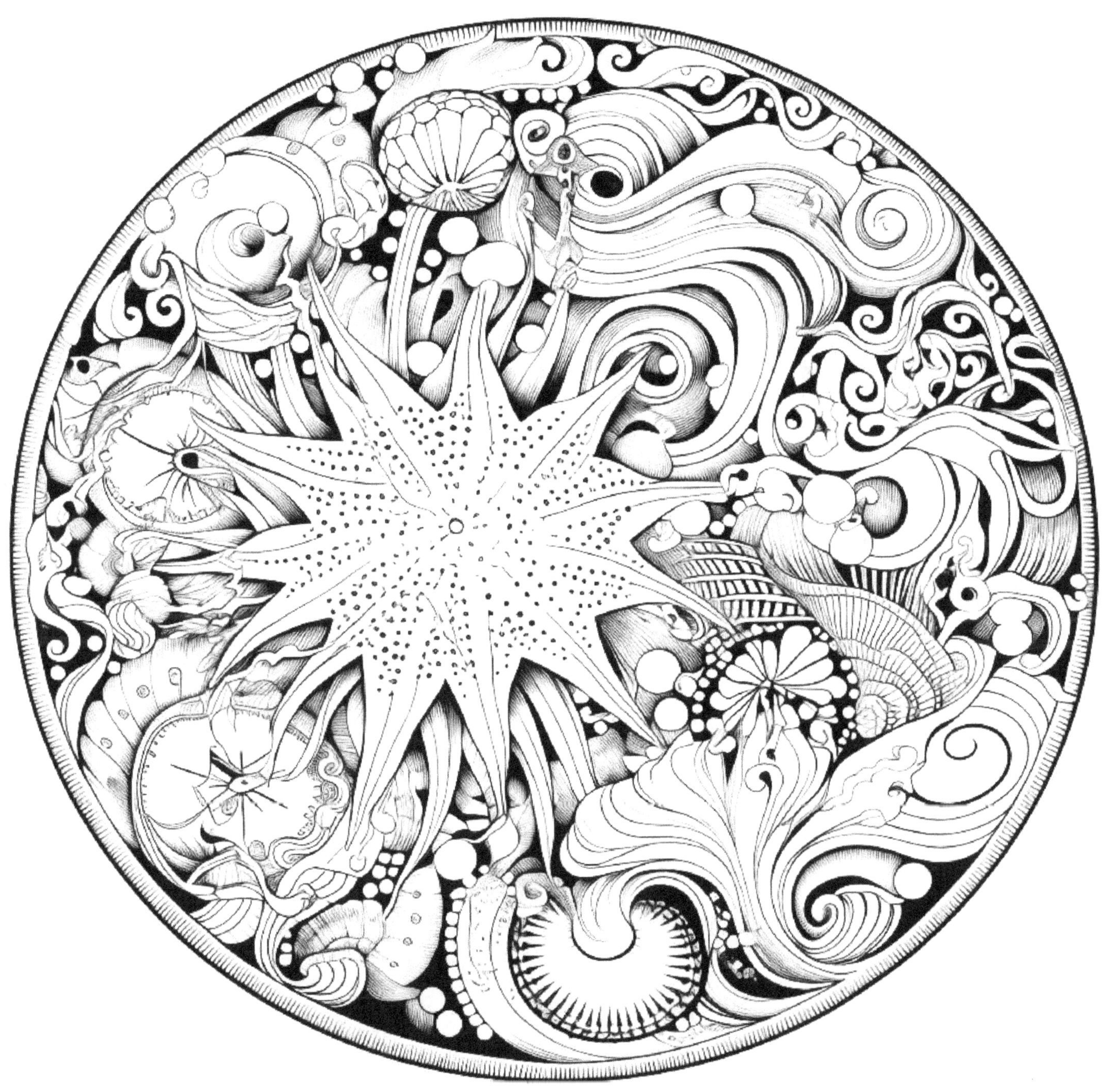

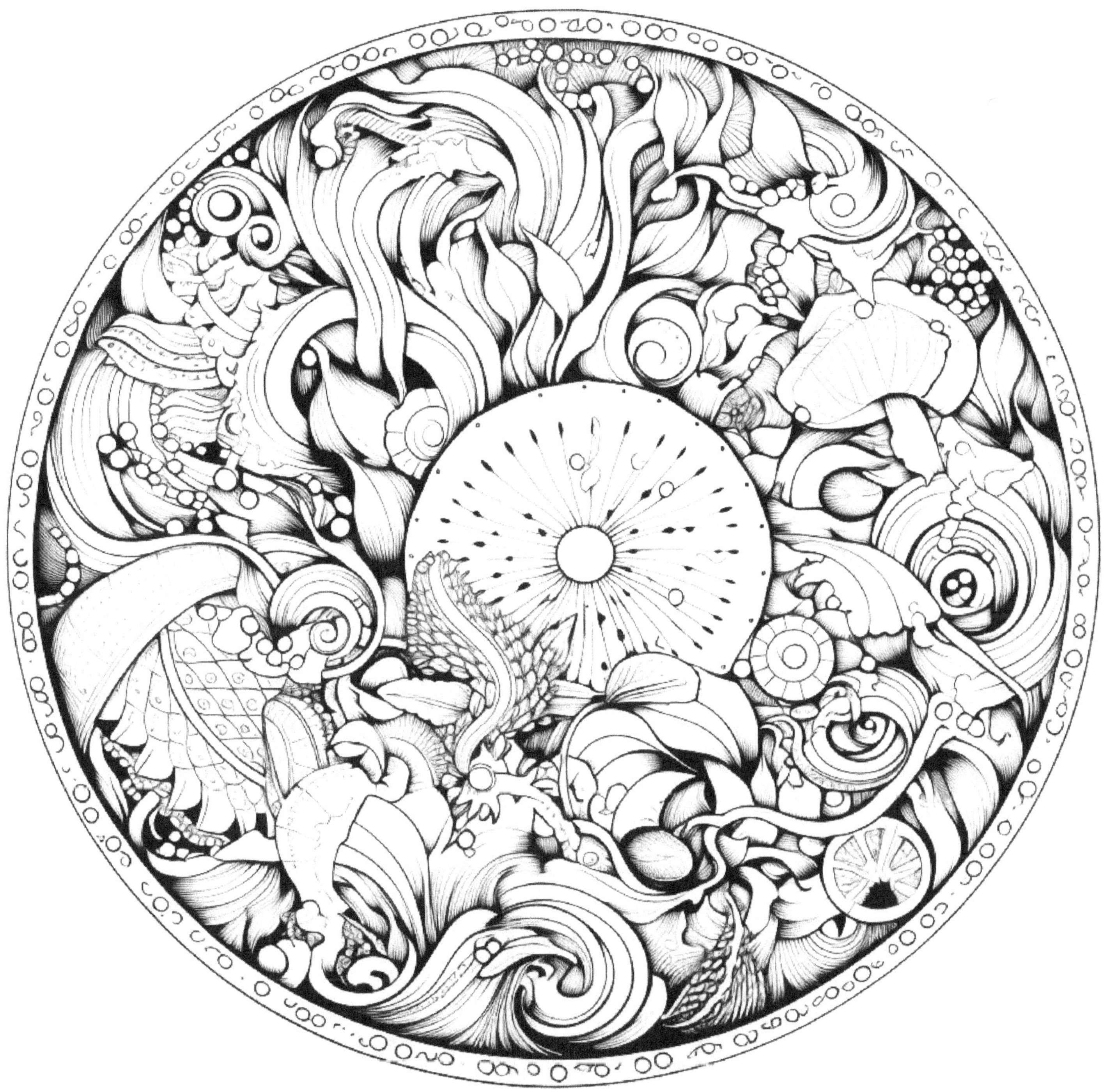

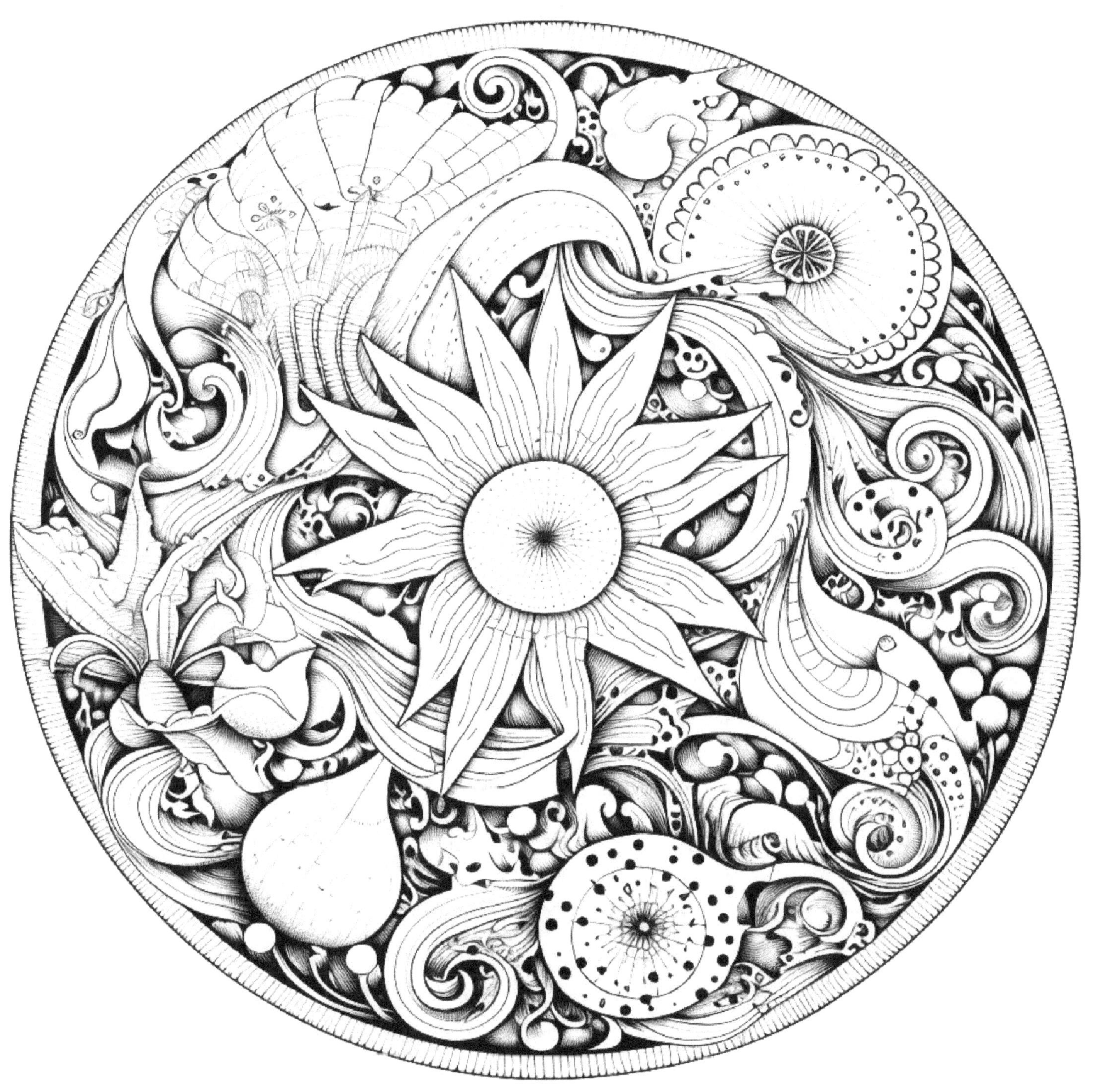

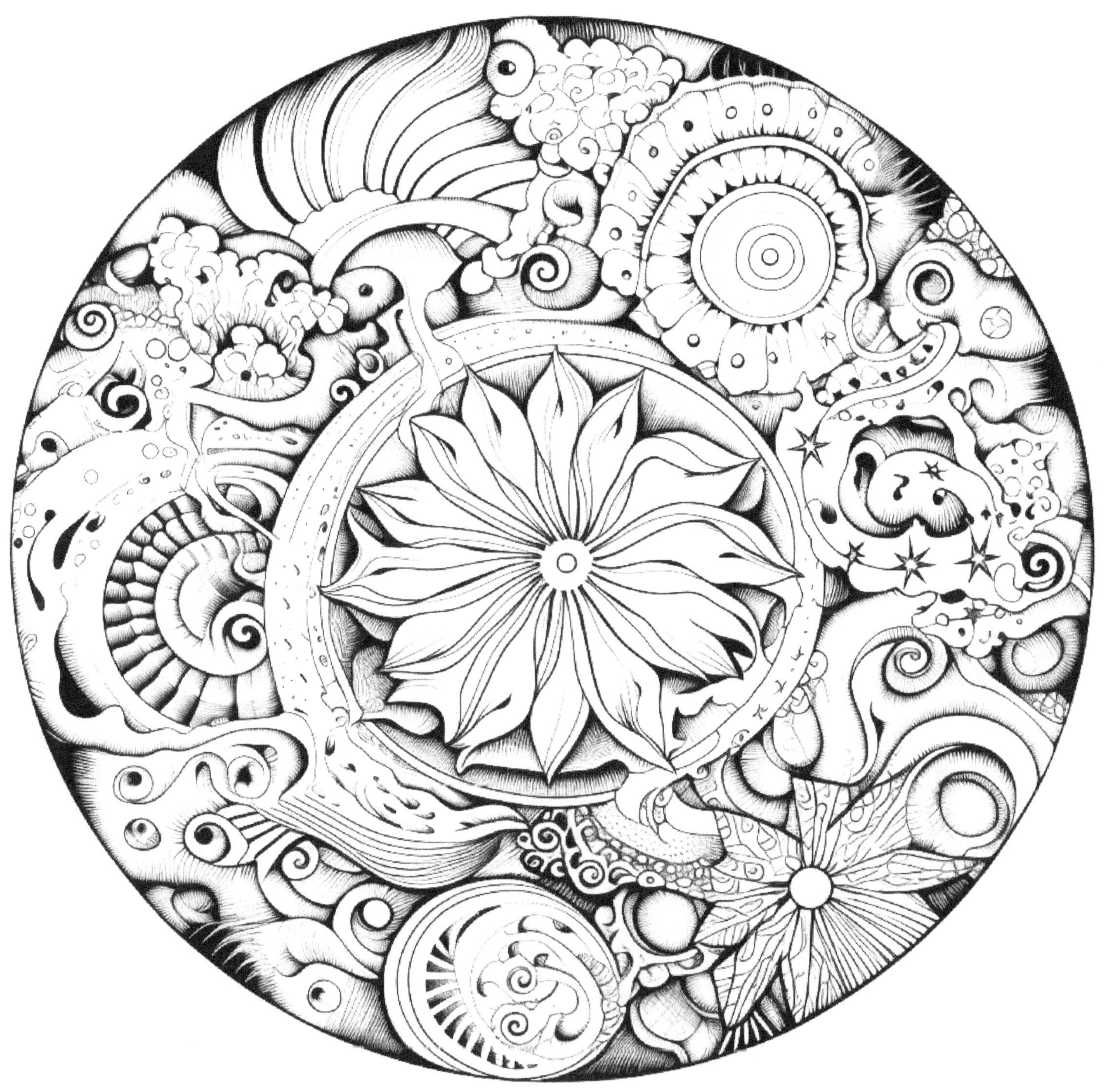

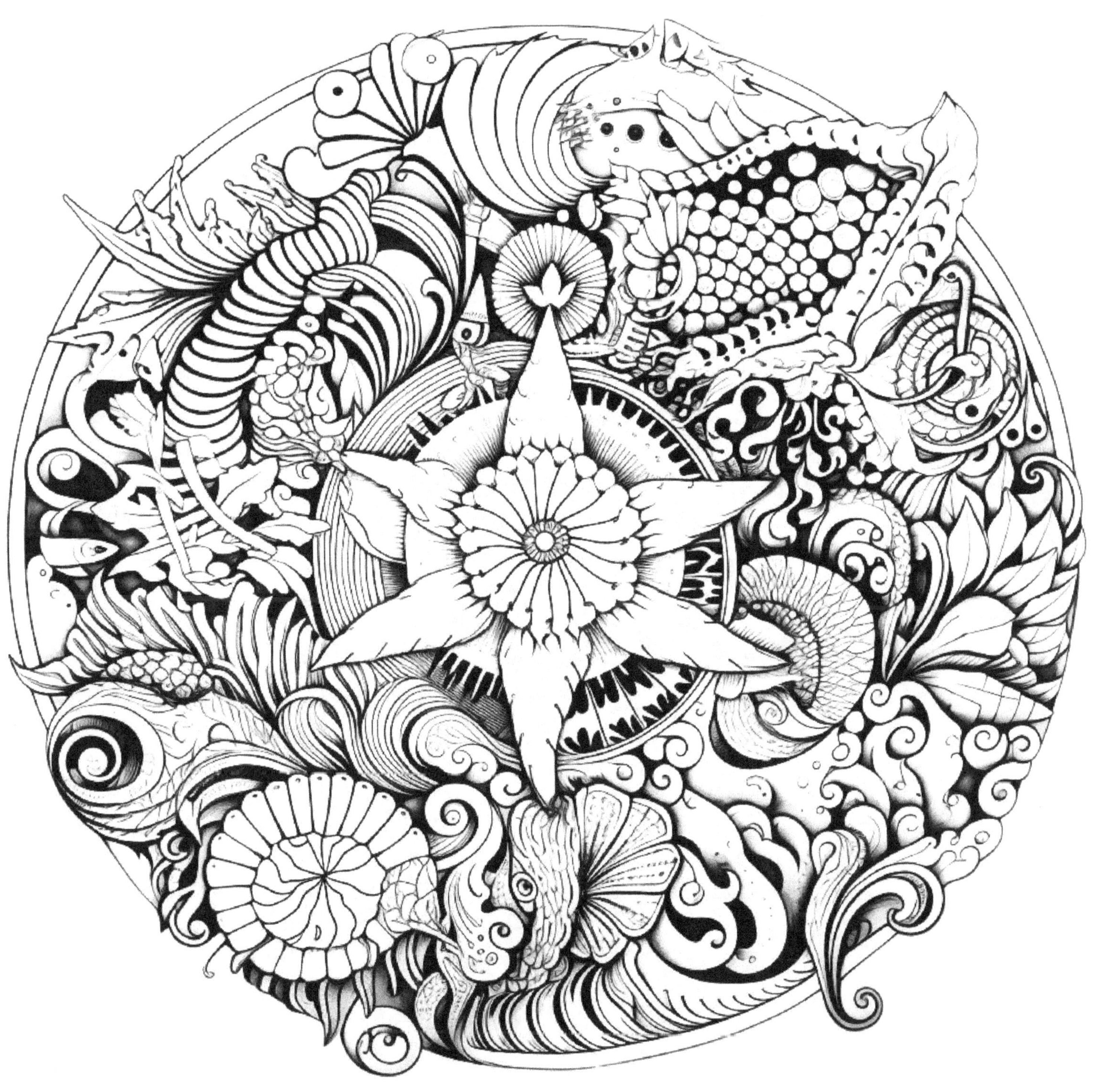

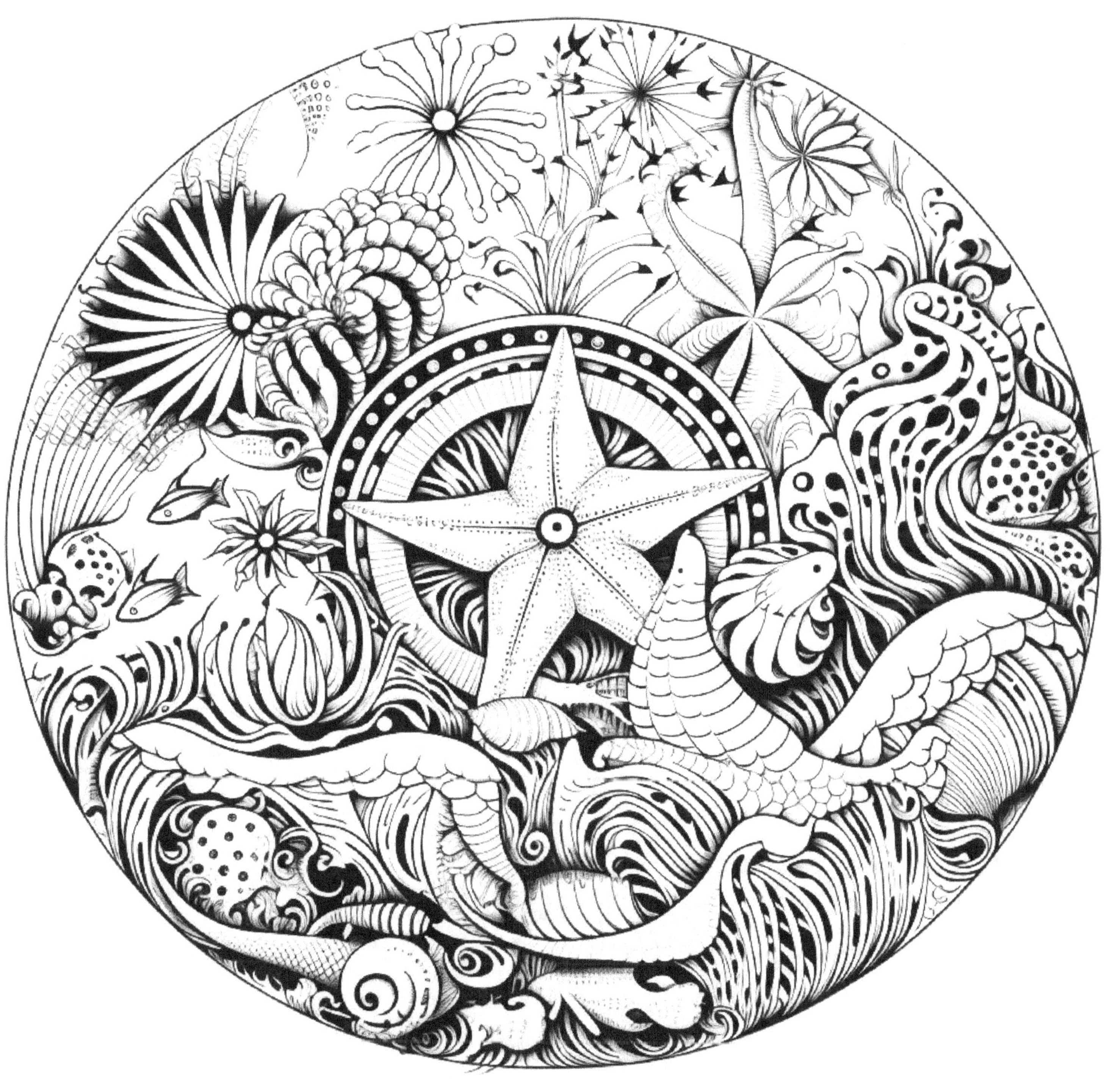

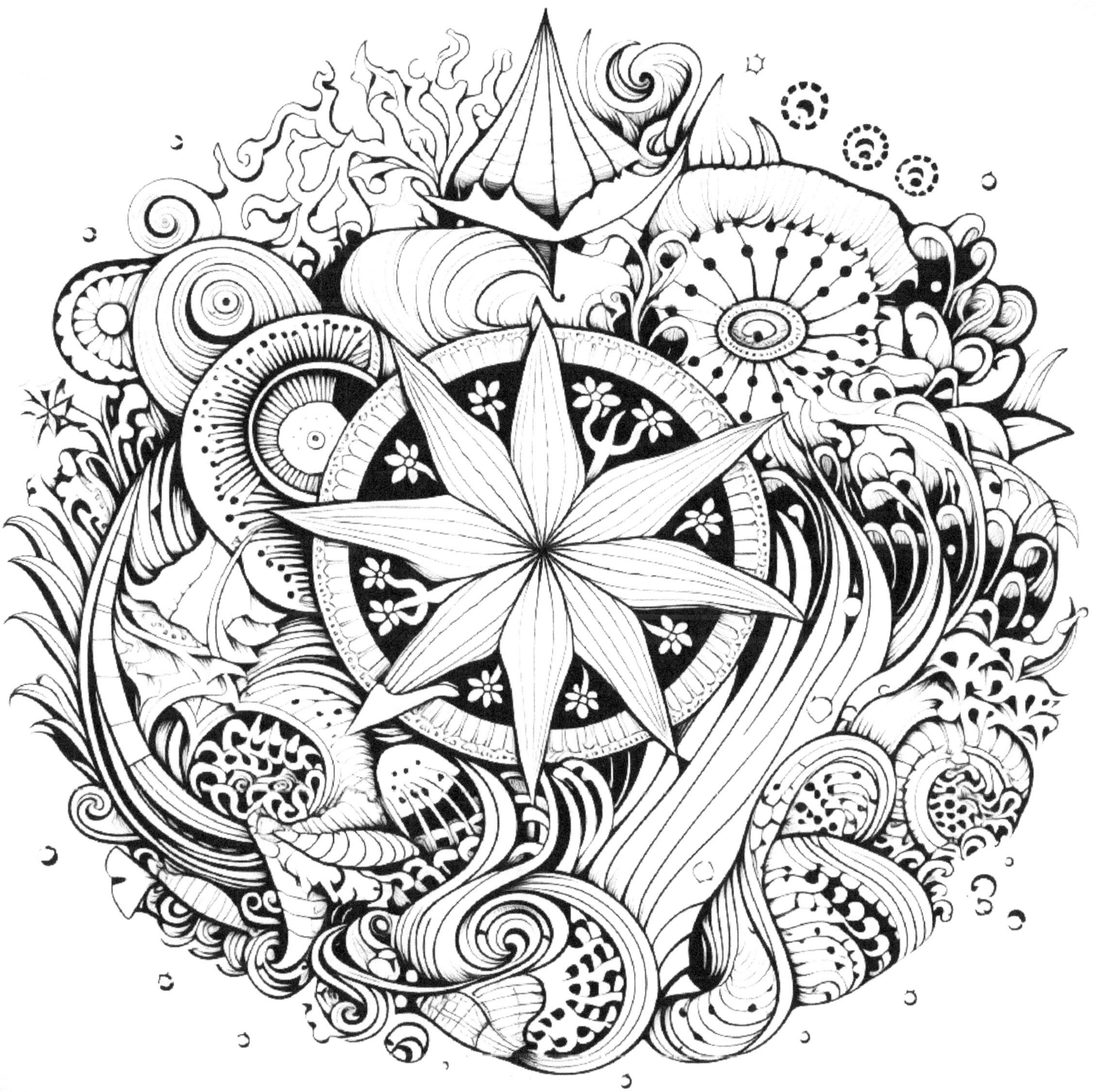

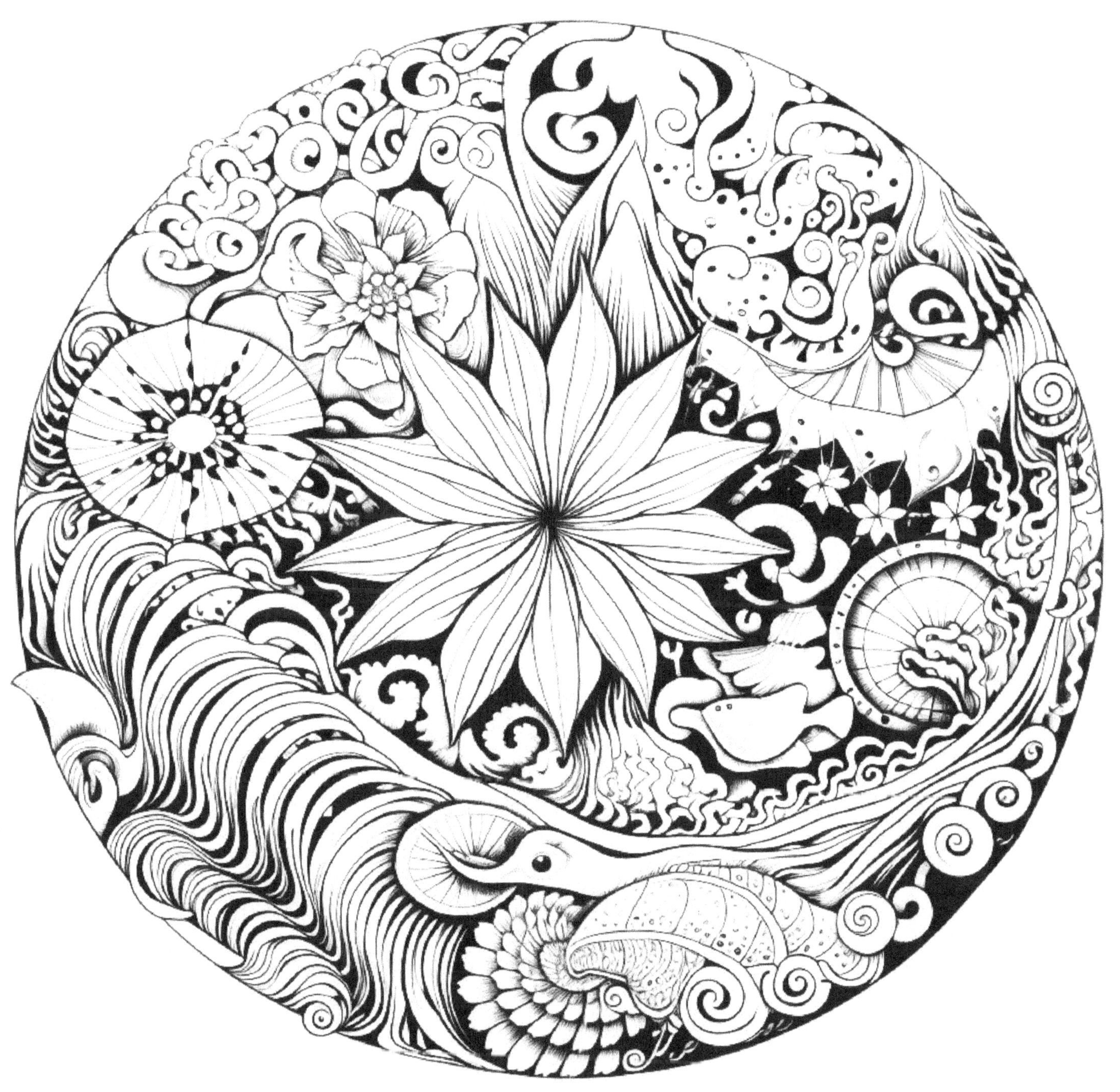

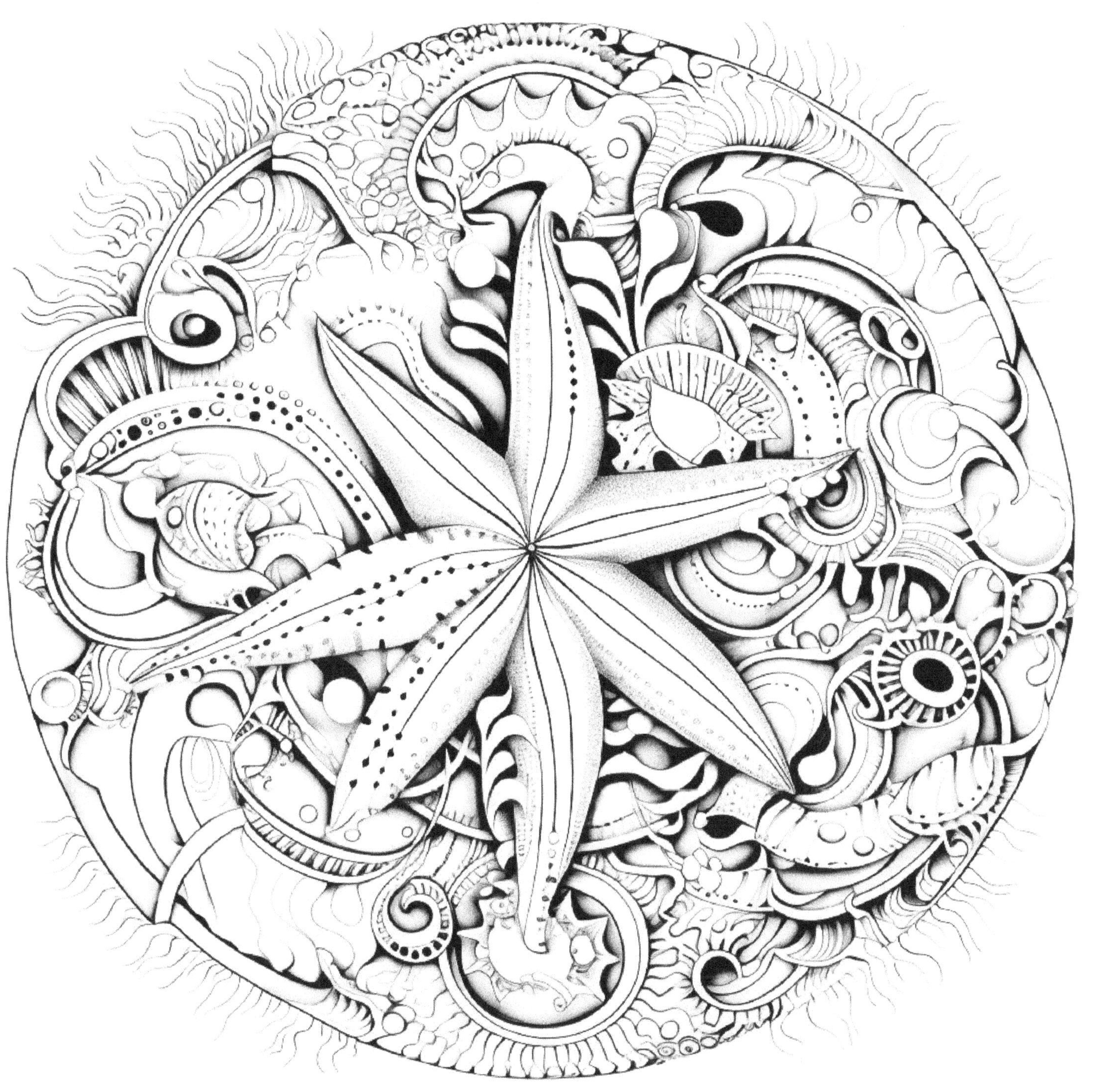

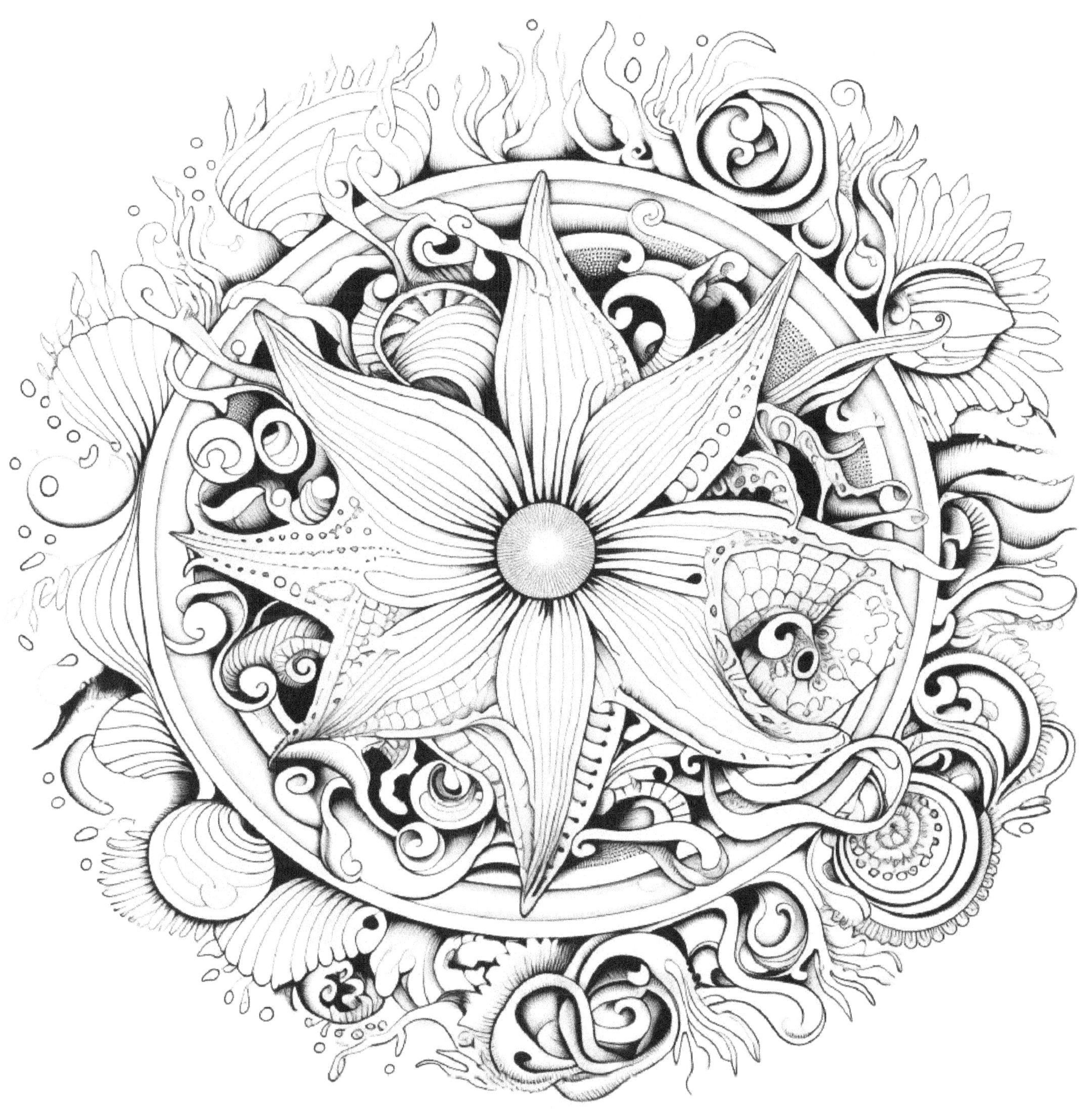

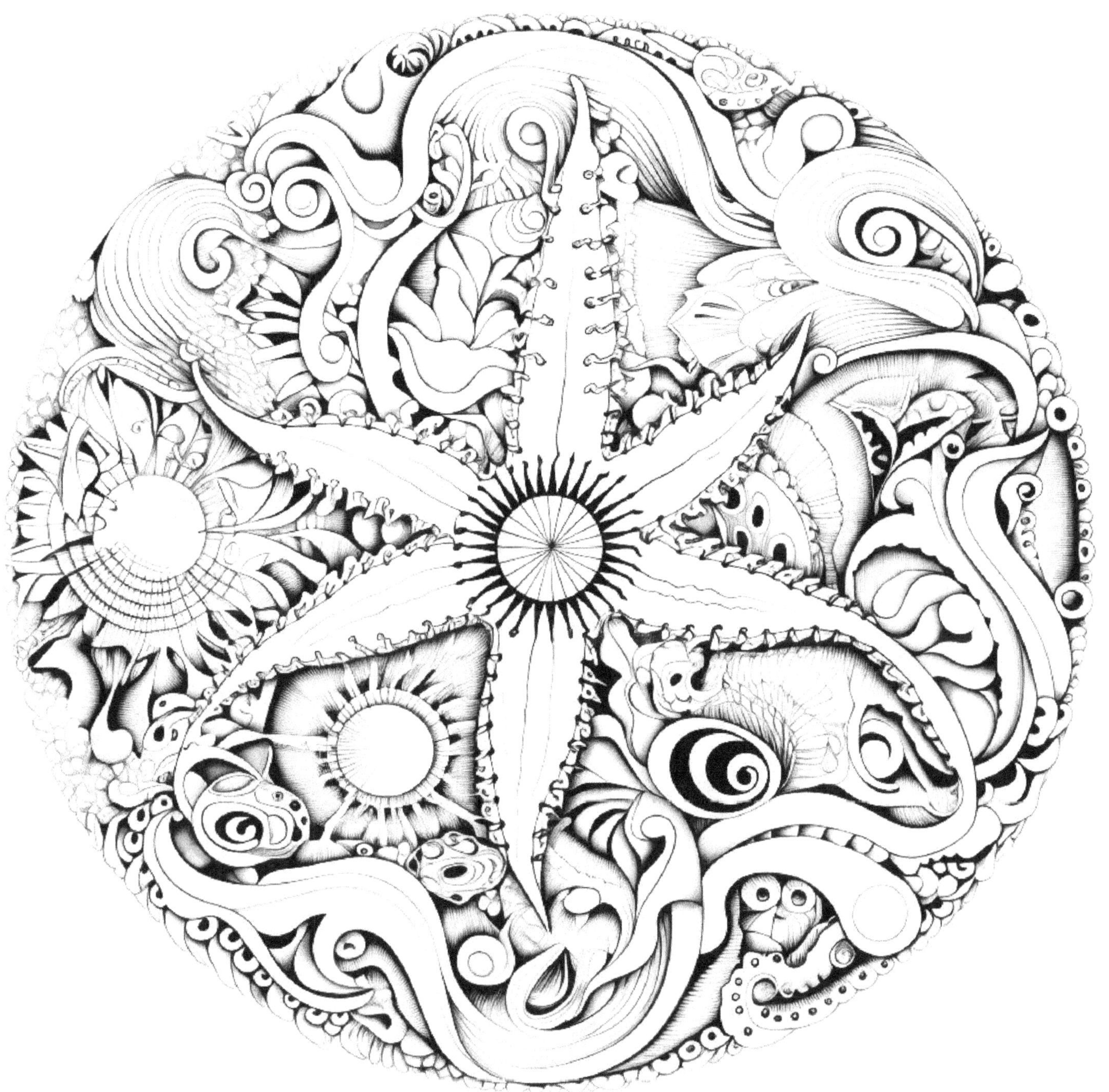

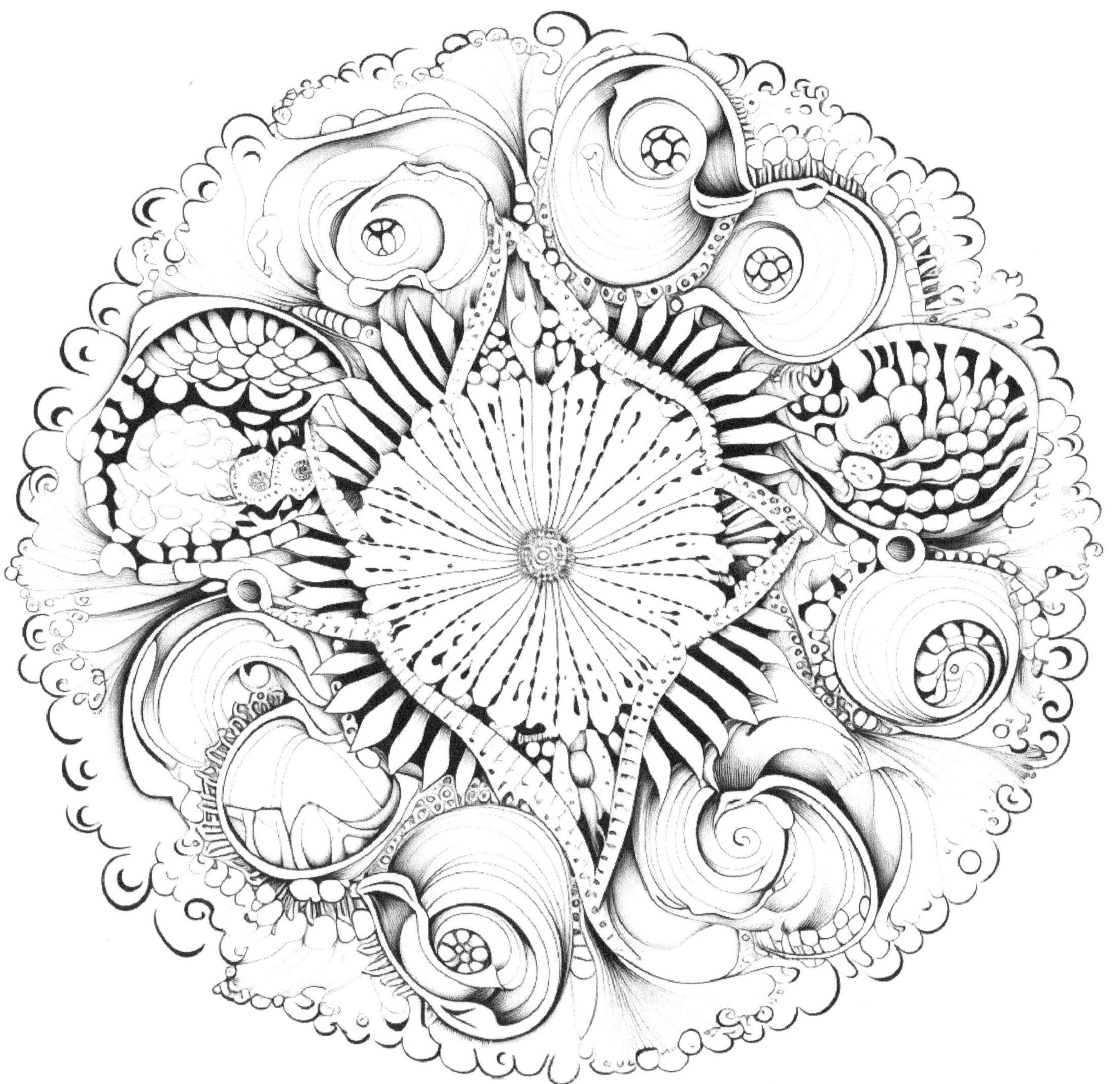

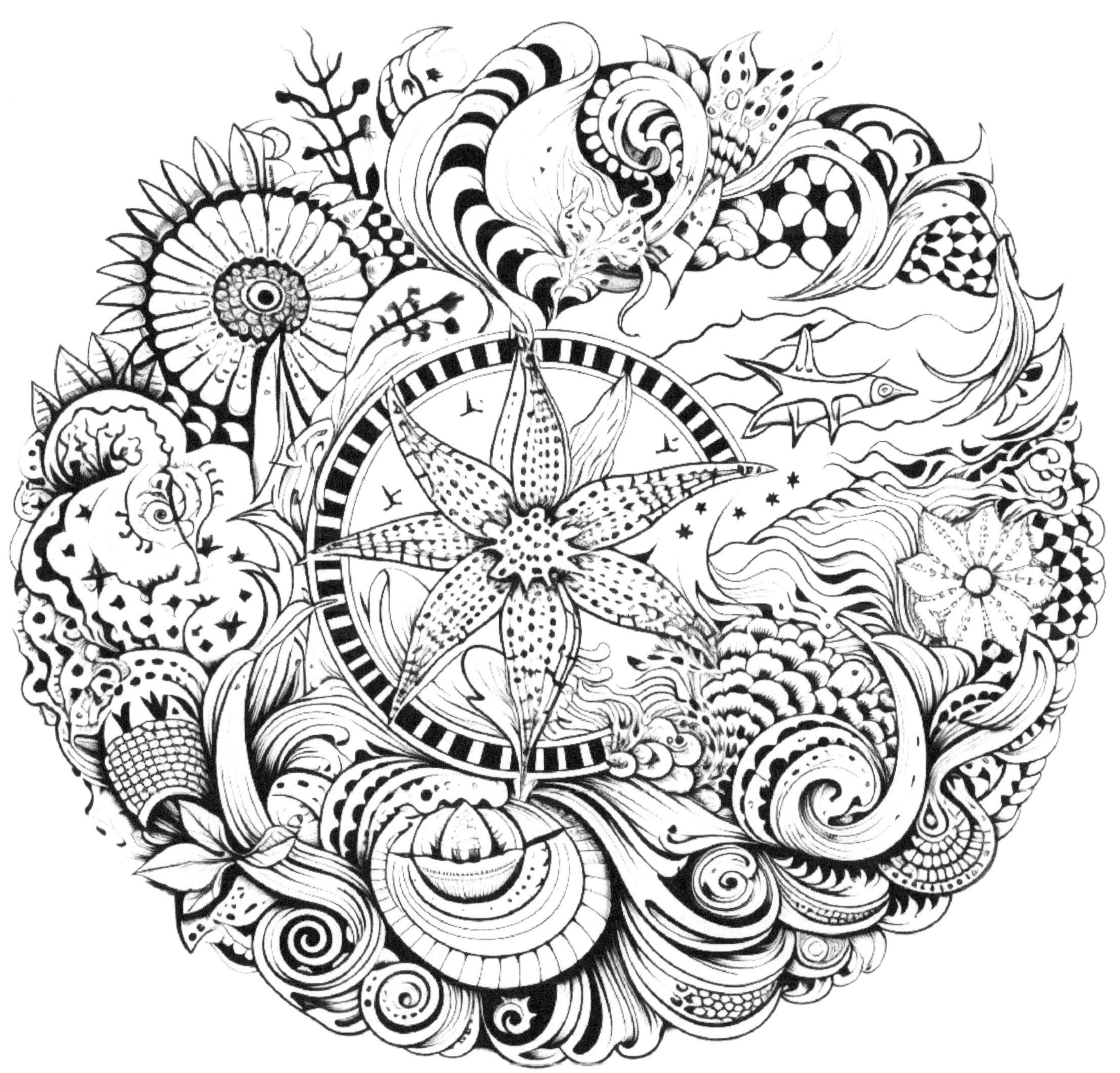

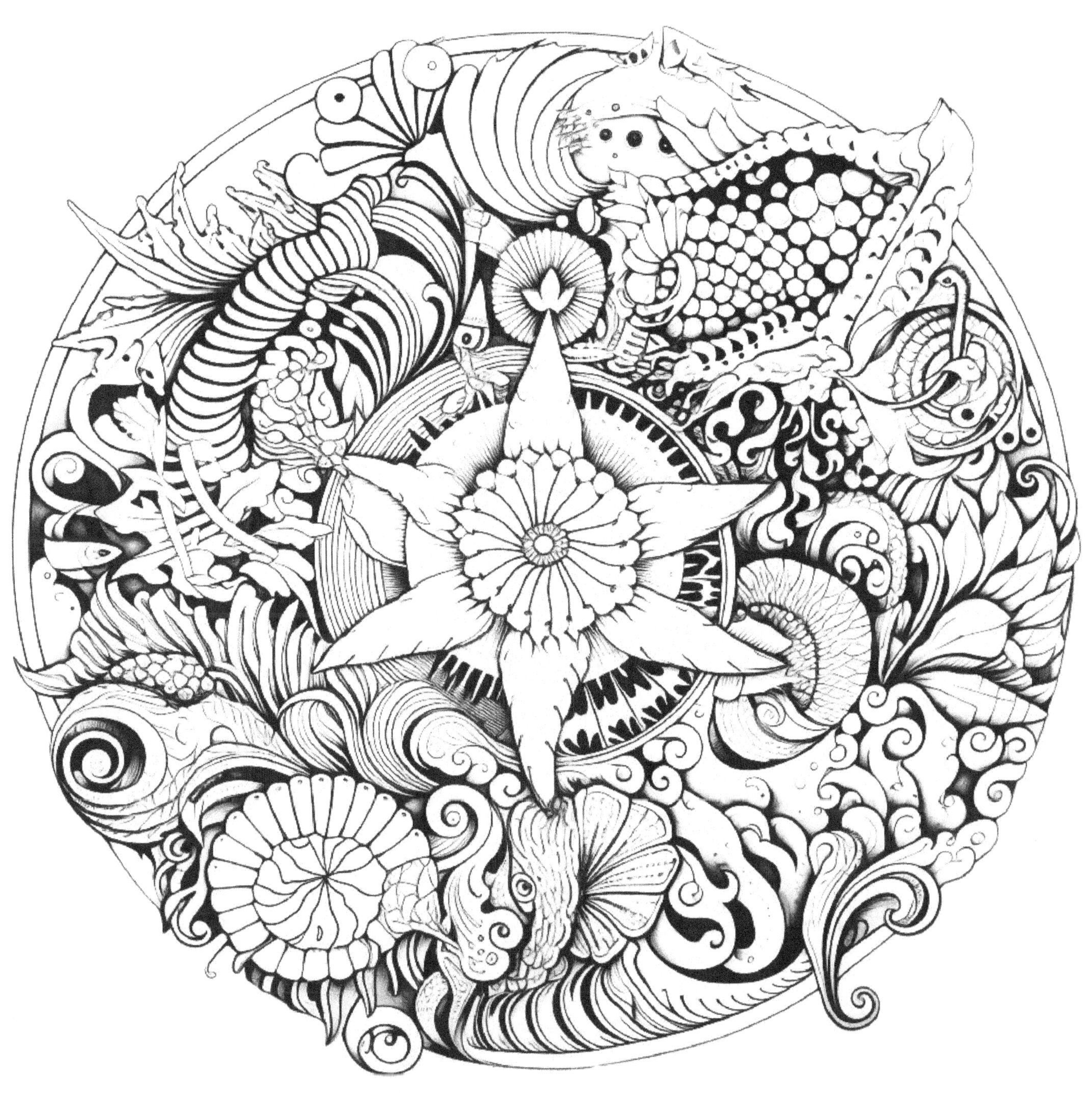

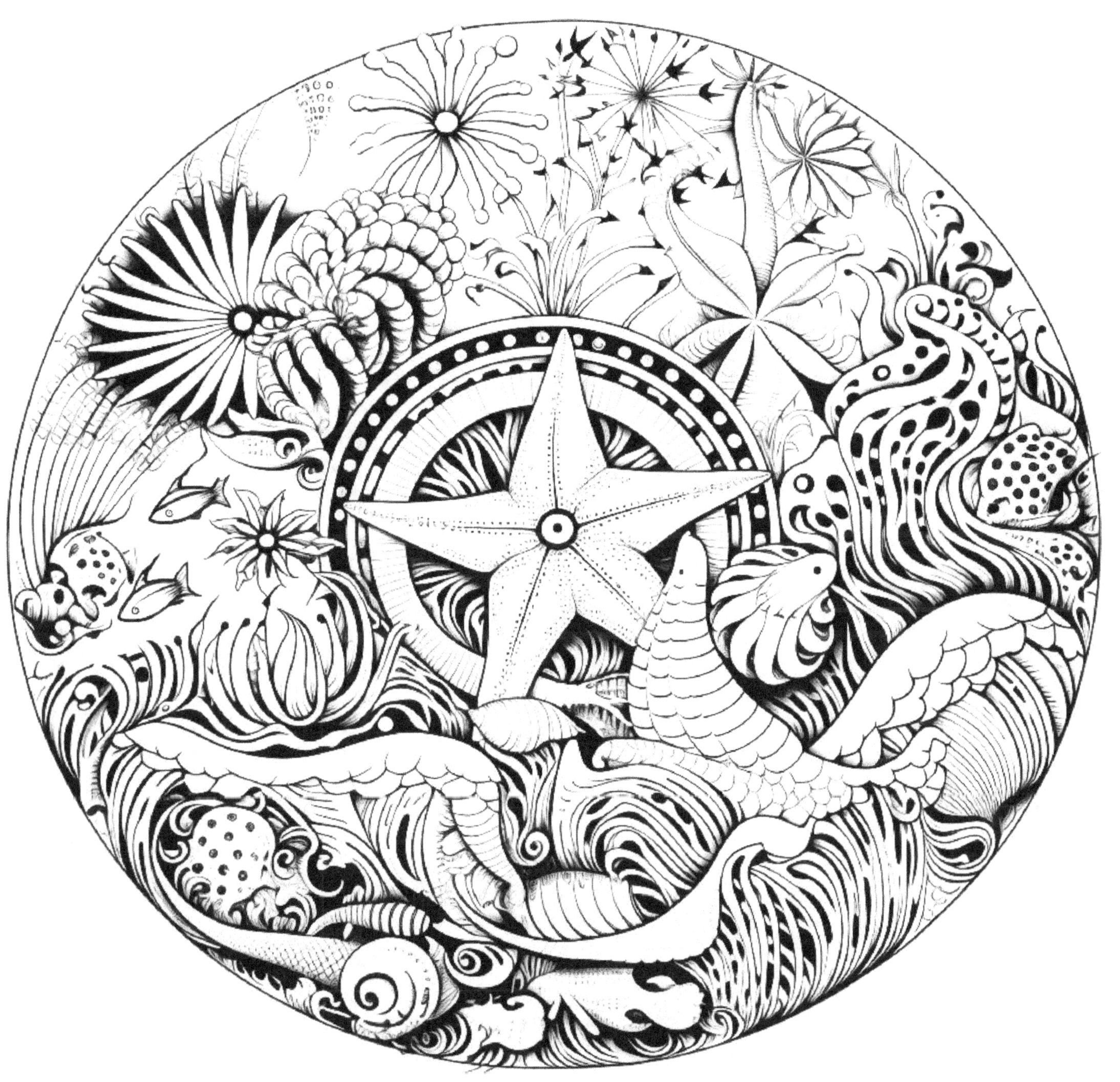

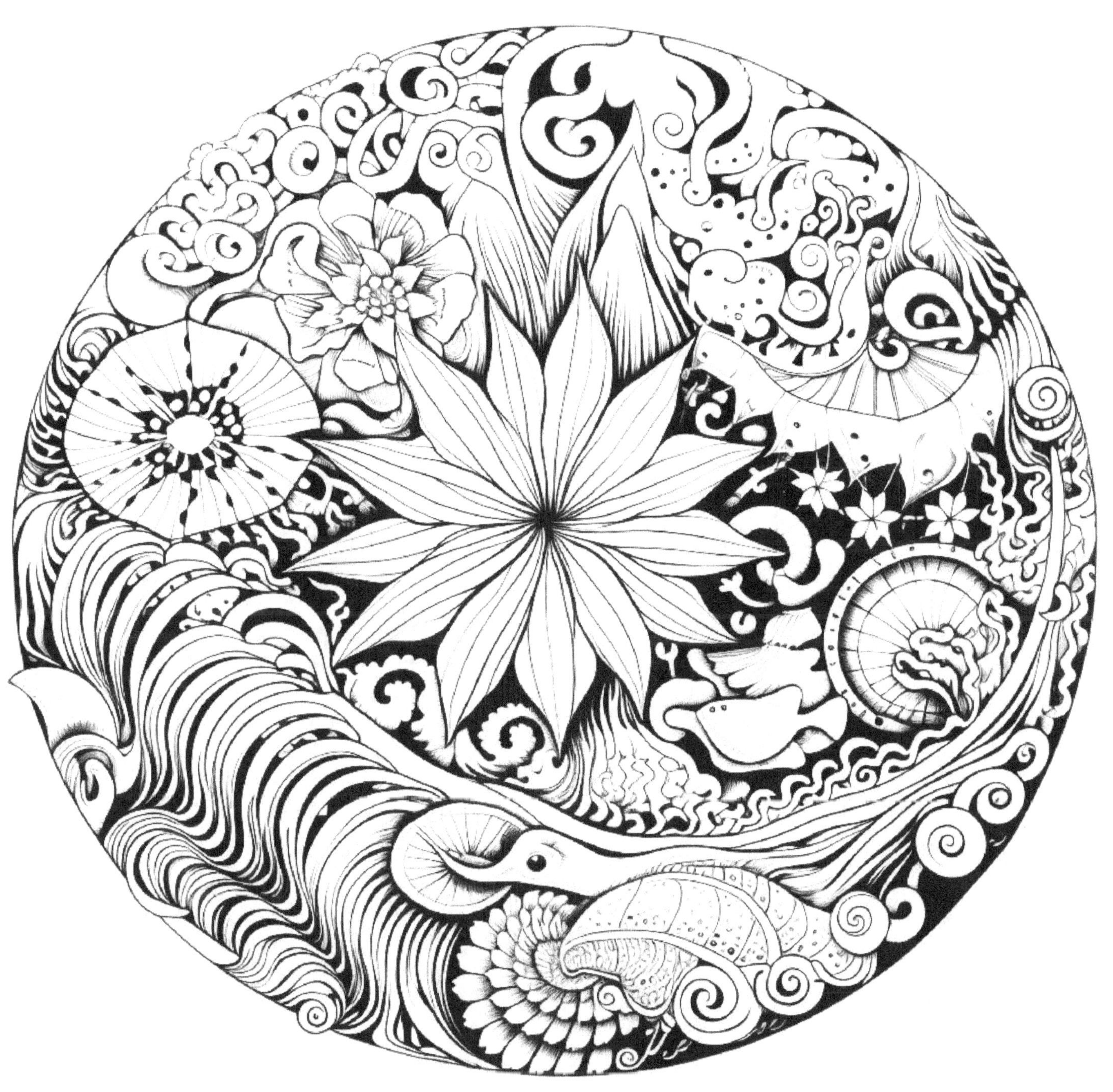

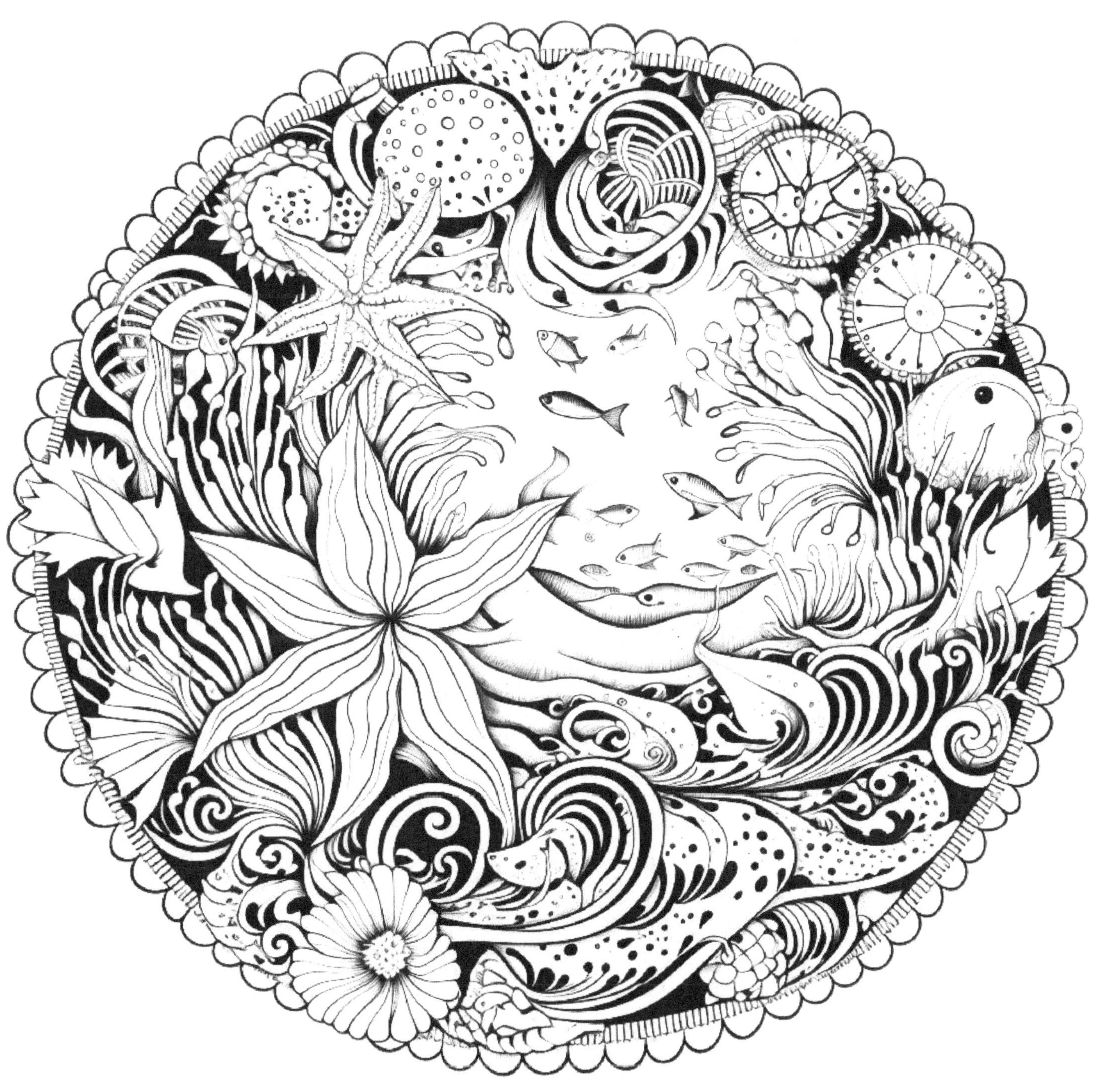

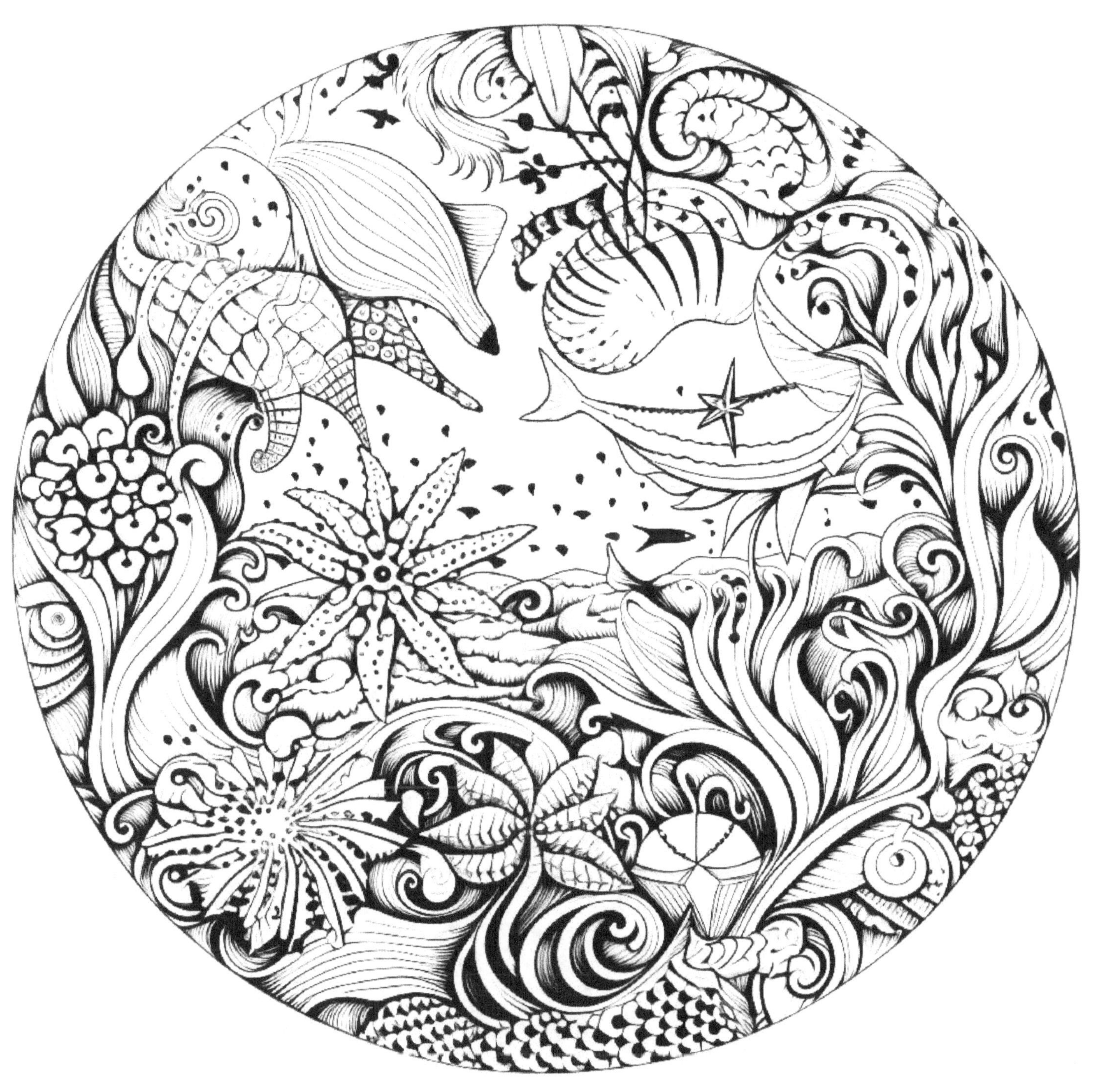

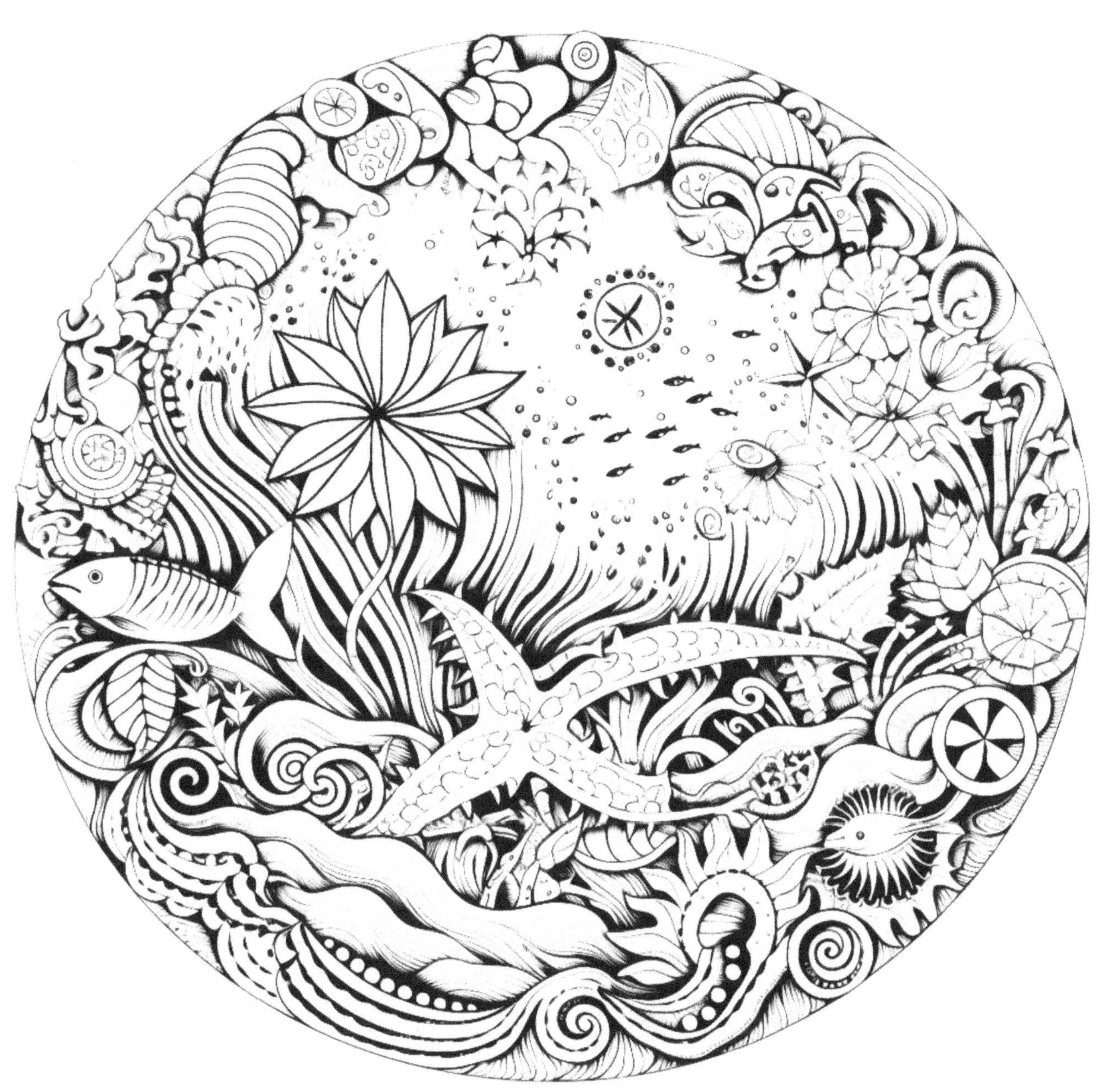

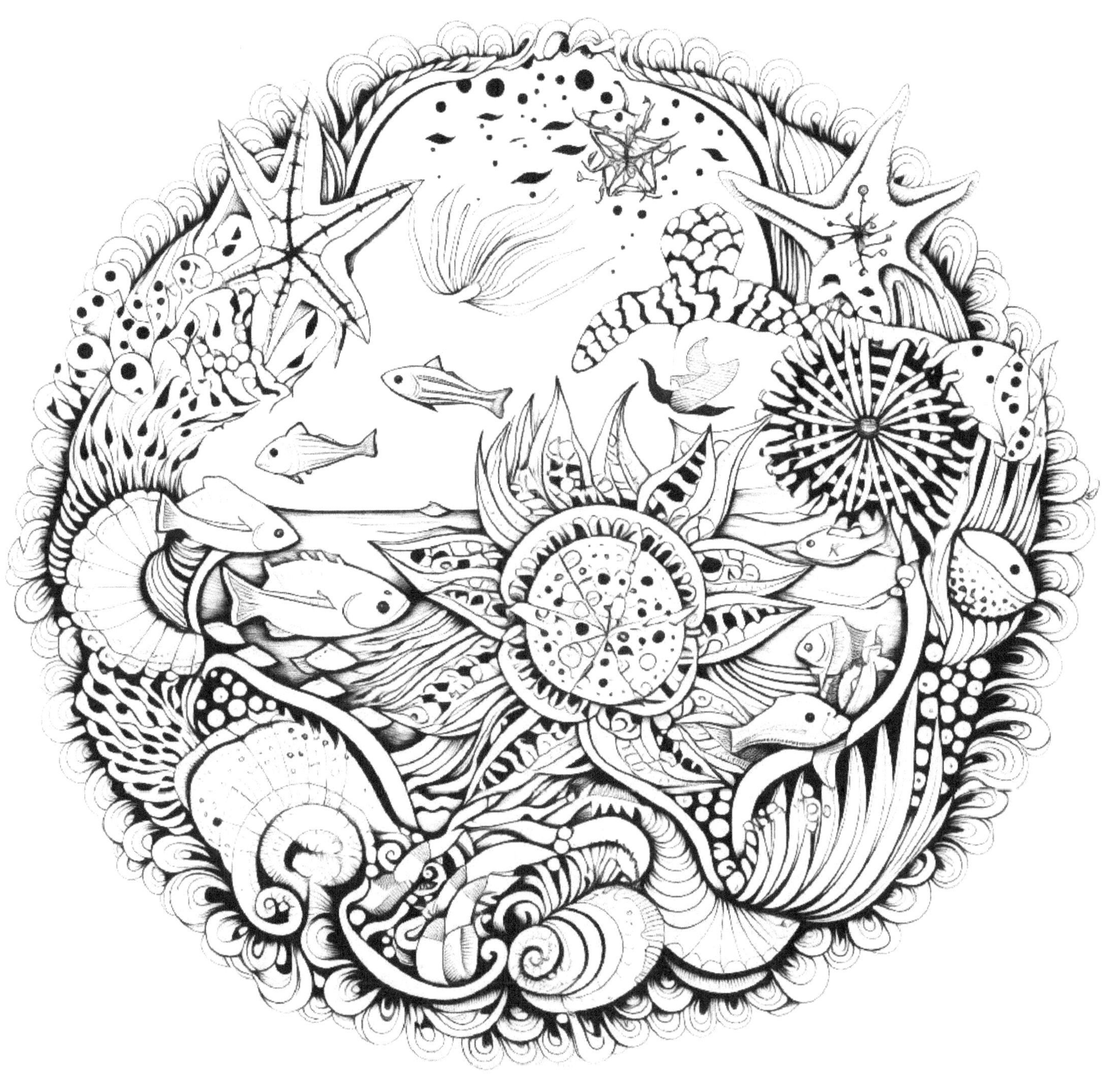

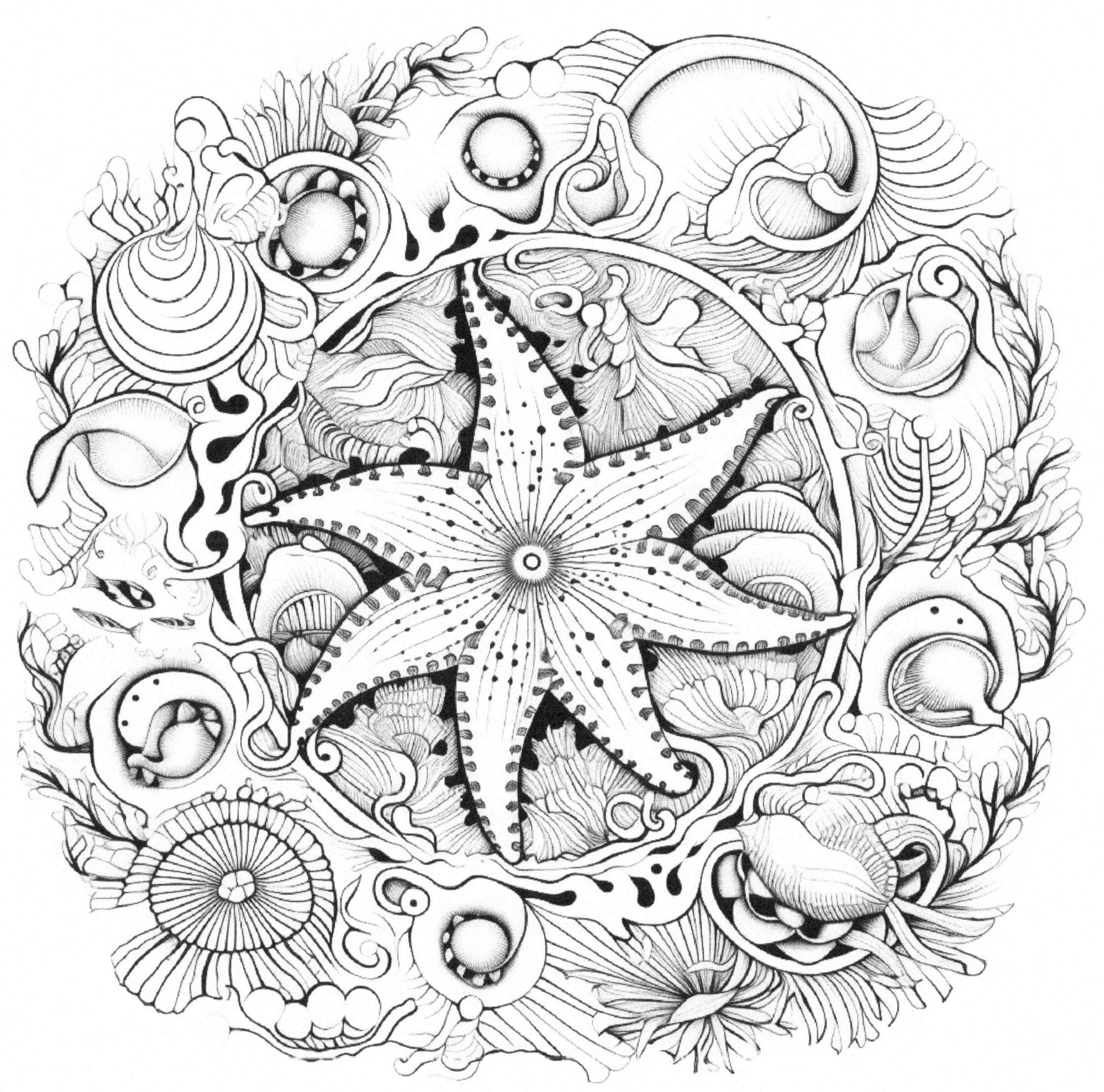

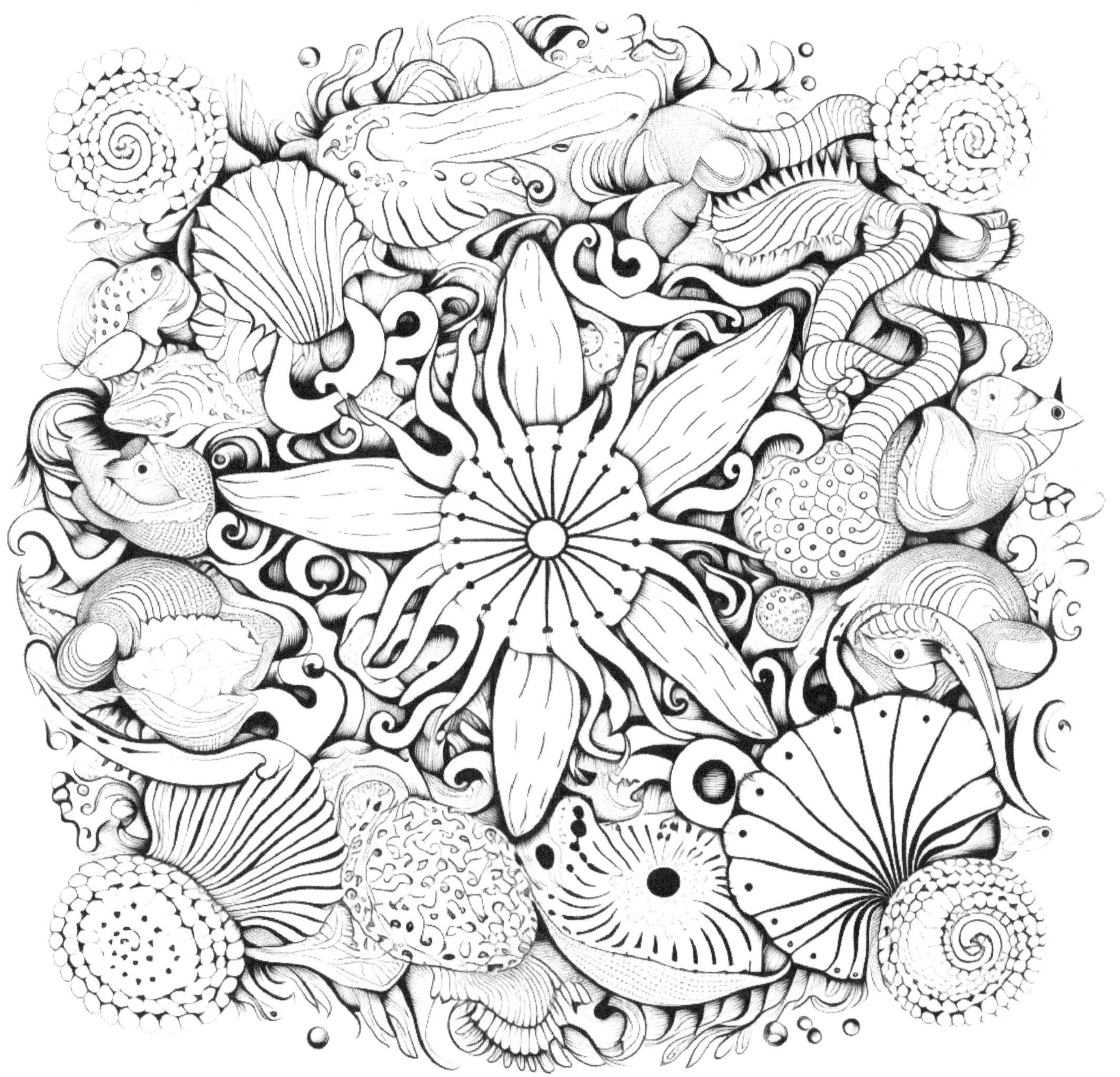

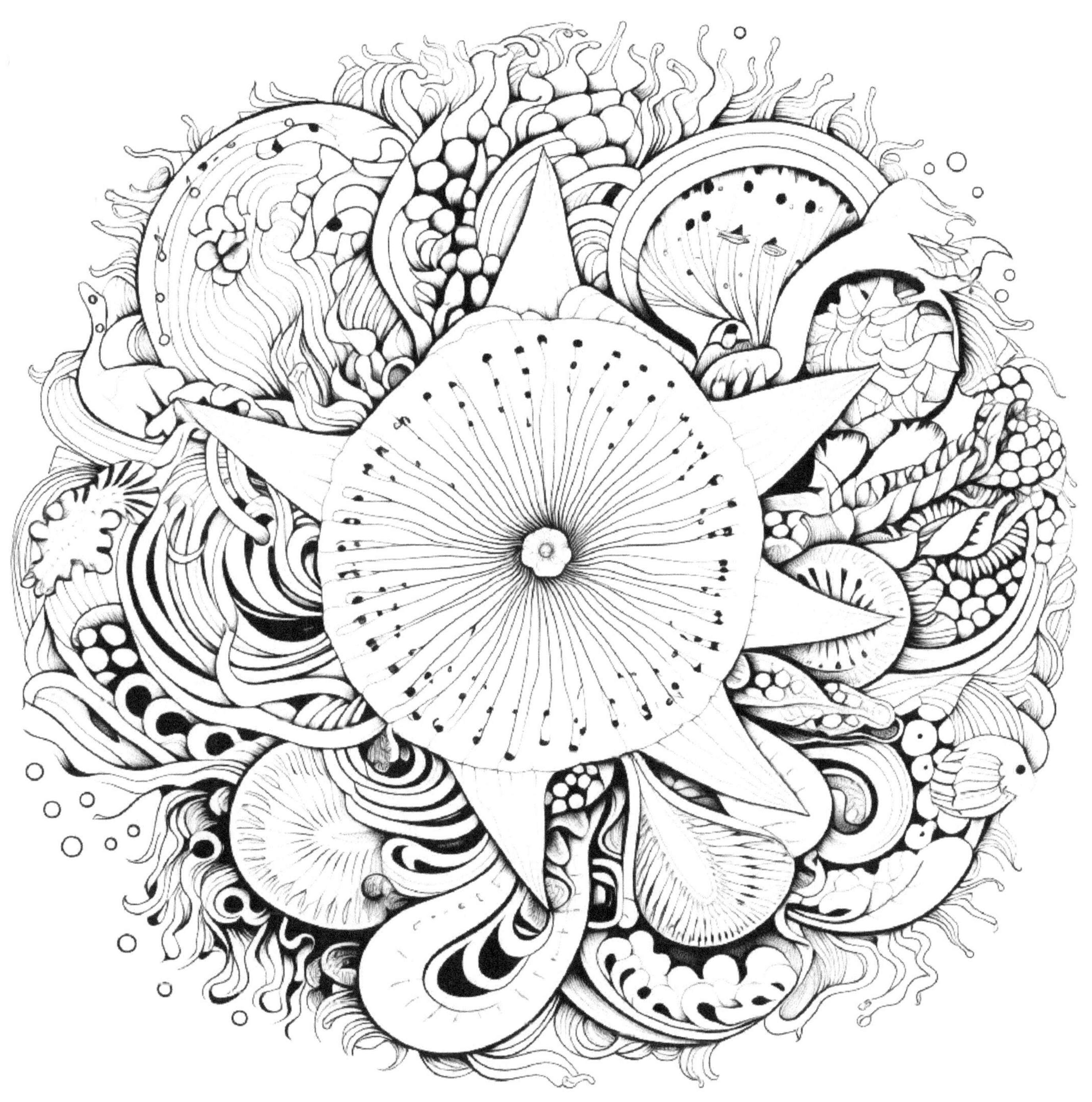

THANK YOU
FOR
YOUR
SUPPORT

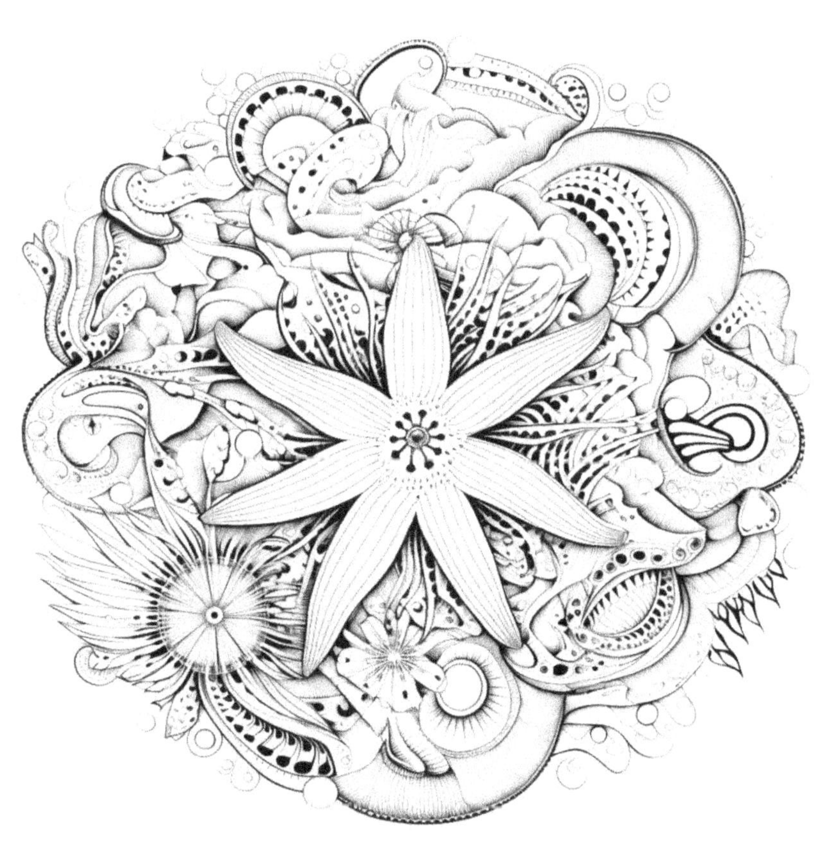

www.ingramcontent.com/pod-product-compliance
Lightning Source LLC
Chambersburg PA
CBHW080919260726
48661CB00009B/3734